The 9 Laws of Health

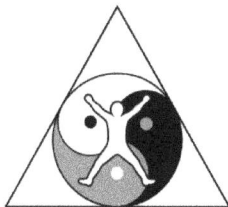

Key to Wellbeing
Grow Healthier - Live Smarter
Live Longer

Christopher Vakas

Foreword by Bob Proctor

Wellbeing Management – Brisbane QLD

WellbeingManagement.com.au

Ordering Information & Quantity Sales: Special discounts are available for quantity purchases by corporations, associations and other groups. For details contact the publisher at: publisher@wm.com.au

Title: The 9 Laws of Health

Subtitle: Key to Wellbeing, Grow Healthier - Live Smarter - Live Longer

Author: Christopher Vakas

Editor: Jill Antuar

First Printed Edition, 2020

ISBN: 978 0648973 11 9

*This book is dedicated to the
doctors, teachers, and mentors who over the years,
have helped me survive and overcome
my own personal health challenges,
so that I could write this book.*

Foreword

I was particularly pleased Christopher Vakas asked me to write the foreword to this book. My whole adult life has been devoted to very similar thinking and information. The fact is, I've been absolutely fascinated with the human personality, what makes us tick and why only a small percentage of the population succeed. I have to agree 100% with Christopher, there are absolute laws that govern each one of us. The fact that he is bringing these laws to us with respect to our health is such a magnificent contribution.

This is, without question, the most comprehensive book on health I've ever gone through. The book is unique in many different respects. It is not just based on knowledge; it is actually based on experience. I'd like you to consider the difference between the two. Knowledge may be something you have learned through some form of study. Experience, however, is something you've done. It's not just something you think is correct, you know it is.

Christopher Vakas had an extraordinary near-death experience. To say he was sick would be an understatement, he truly was very close to dying. He sought and found advice on what he could do, and he found out if he was going to enjoy any health, it would be something he would have to do, not anybody else. Doctors prescribing various drugs was not going to solve his problem. He followed what many would consider an almost impossible regimen, and he did get better. He also became fascinated with the body.

In his own words, he stated, "Over the past 28 years I have searched for the secrets to health and well-being, spent years researching medical journals, and studying health science to gain a better understanding on how the environment can impact heath. I've read well over 100 books, trolled though countless studies, articles, reports, and critical trials to bring you the truth of the laws that govern health and have been here all along."

I have been in the personal development business for going on sixty years, and like Christopher, I have read hundreds of books, studied numerous articles and rarely take my mind off of the subject of how we can enjoy a greater quality of life. I, too, have become fascinated as to why people do what they do, and why they do not do many of the things they know they should do.

To bring our attention back to the laws again, Dr. Werhner Von Braun, who was considered the father of the space program, stated the natural laws of the universe are so precise that we have no problem building spaceships, sending people to the moon and we can time the landing with the precision of a half a second. What Christopher is offering in this book is how those laws apply to our life and why they must be followed if we want to enjoy a healthy life.

This book has my attention; I intend to keep reading it. In fact, I intend to study it. And I believe after you've read it you will feel indebted to the author as much as I do. This is definitely a book you should share with your friends. The content will make incredible discussion material.

Bob Proctor, Teacher in The Secret and Bestselling Author of You Were Born Rich.

Author's Note

If you are suffering from a degenerative disease, are tired all the time, seem to get every cold or flu going around, have an immune disorder or simply want to attain your ideal weight and be healthier, consult and work with your doctor or health care professional as you read this book, so they can monitor and observe your progress. If your doctor is dismissive of the truths expounded by this book, you need to find another doctor.

Both you and your doctor will be astonished by the rapid healing and newfound health that will result as you live these nine laws daily. Visits to the doctor will become less frequent over time, and only be required for check-ups or injuries that require immediate medical attention.

Disclaimer

Certain information contained in this book is derived from sources that Christopher Vakas and Webmall Pty Ltd believe to be reliable; however, we do not guarantee the accuracy or timeliness of the information and assume no liability for any resulting damages. Readers should seek advice from their doctor or health care professional regarding the appropriateness of the information referred to within this book for their particular situation. Christopher Vakas is not a practising Doctor of Medicine.

Table of Contents

Prologue

It is time for a new philosophy on wellbeing. I look around and am appalled at the poor level of health of the masses. People are sicker and heavier than they ought to be and our hospitals are overflowing. At any time of the day or night you can visit the accident and emergency section of any hospital and you will see there an ever-growing group that visits for completely preventable illnesses. To be sure you will see people who have been injured and require immediate medical care; but it is the first group, who are getting sick when they ought not to be, that this book is for.

If you want to shed weight naturally, get fitter naturally, have an abundance of energy all day every day, live longer and feel great, this book is for you. I am not going to go into the preventable illnesses in great detail in this book, as they are just that, preventable. This is a book about how to understand and apply the laws that govern health. These laws have always been here and you no doubt will be familiar with some, if not all, of them to some extent. The essence is, therefore, how easily they can be learnt and applied to attain optimum health, ideal weight, wellbeing, mental and physical fitness and to keep it throughout your life?

Our health and wellbeing are, to a great extent, controlled by our desires for health, for it all starts with desire. This is usually the easy bit, as we all want to be healthy. It is our beliefs that either stop us or keep us on the right track when the going gets tough; and you can count on it that it will, at least initially, with some of the lifestyle changes that may be needed.

If you feel you lack belief in yourself, you can have belief in the principles outlined in this book; for they will never let you down, if you use them. It is ok if at first you are struggling with some of these nine laws for health, as most people do initially. If you persist and increase your awareness and understanding of how these laws operate to govern health, you will succeed.

The purpose of this book is to give you the simple truths and the laws that govern health and lifelong wellbeing, along with some of the activities that will get you there. The nine laws of health described in this book could be summed up in a paragraph; however, that would deprive the reader of the awareness that comes from understanding the principles behind the laws. All the gloss and fluff has been removed so that the nine prerequisites for health are easy to follow for anyone who truly wants to be healthy.

You might be thinking, "Is it possible to maintain vibrant health in a world filled with conflicting information purported to be the truth?" There are companies promoting products that appear so miraculous that once consumed, will magically give you a new body at its ideal weight, with perfect health and longevity. The truth is our health is governed by exacting laws, and it really will not matter what products we consume if we are violating the laws. The products may be great to enhance and support a person living in harmony with the laws, but these products will never replace the very basic nine prerequisites described in this book.

Many great scientists have employed scientific methods to test theories and hypotheses regarding the cause of disease, hopeful cures, what is good for you, what is bad for you, what to eat and what to avoid. Unfortunately, many scientific studies are funded by pharmaceutical companies or fast-food manufacturers. Scientific methods will tell you what is not true, what cannot be proved or what could be; however, it cannot arrive at an absolute truth. There is good reason for this. Science is evolving. What appears to be established and proven, is only as good as the methods employed to arrive at the conclusions drawn. For example, scientific methods employ representative controls and cohorts of samples that are all believed to be representative of the study and hypothesis being tested. However, are all the variables being considered? When one is dealing with the human body, the variables are as infinite as the number of people living on the planet. Further, the complexity of the human body, the physical and social environment, genetic history, and diversity suggest that conclusions drawn by scientific methods alone are, at best, inadequate.

Despite all the confusion out there, there have been hundreds of years of quality research funded by taxpayers like you and me. Most, if not all governments expend taxpayer funds to commission research from the world's most trusted research institutions. This research is published in the most respected scientific journals globally. Once understood, they paint a very clear picture of the truths that you will find in this book regarding which choices tend to improve health and wellbeing, and which choices tend to lead to disease.

The degradation of our environment places increasing pressure on the body's ability to satisfy what we can call external natural environmental health needs, of which there are three. We will get into these a bit later in the book. Other significant influencers include our biological physical needs – again there are three. Another is our genetic makeup, which may go back many generations. Additionally, there are complex social environments, where positive and negative influences shape our beliefs and values. This genetic disposition and social influence are what we will call the learned habitual influences that are driven largely by the subconscious mind. These can be broadly categorised as psychological needs – again there are three.

Interestingly, this past fifty years, I, along with a host of other great scientists and thinkers, have observed that there is an increasing number of people getting sick and dying of preventable diseases. You would expect this to some extent, because there are billions more people on the planet since the 'Father of Medicine' Hippocrates (460-377 BC) walked the earth. Although he only lived until eighty-three, he knew a thing or two about the laws of health. At his time there were only around 100 million people in total on the planet, and not many lived past fifty. At the time of writing this book, around 7.8 billion people live on this planet and we now know a great deal more about what it takes to enjoy lifelong health. Many of the scientists whose work I refer to in this book are concerned with this preventable disease scourge that is afflicting humanity, after having observed our hospitals getting bigger, in direct proportion to the waistline of the population. Cognitive issues, respiratory and cardiovascular disease, suicide, and social dysfunction are at unprecedented levels, and all types of cancers are on the rise.

One would have to ask, "Why?" There is now so much knowledge available – medical and scientific research and expertise; advances in technology and pharmacology; and an abundant availability of nutritious foods. Why are people still so confused? Why are there so many more unhealthy people now than there have ever been? Why can't anyone who wants it, have vibrant health, ideal weight, abundant energy, and longevity? The good news is that these, and many other important questions, are all answered in the pages of this book.

Over the past 28 years I have searched for the secrets to health and wellbeing, spent years researching medical journals and studying health science, to gain a better understanding of how the environment can impact health. I have read well over 100 books and trolled though countless studies, articles, reports, and clinical trials, to bring you the truth of the laws that govern health that have been here all along.

One thing is for sure, as the body reaches and maintains Level 3 utilisation as discussed later in the book, it is able to restore itself to optimum health. This happens by law, the exacting laws that govern wellbeing.

For those who take the time to learn and apply the nine laws governing wellbeing and put these tried and tested concepts and activities presented here to the test, they too will find that they may: enjoy the benefits of vibrant health, attain their ideal weight, and have the abundant energy and longevity that is being experienced by thousands around the world, who know and apply these laws in their everyday lives. The goals and objectives of this book are to demystify health, by simply showing how you can easily and consistently satisfy the nine fundamental laws of health. These fundamentals, if practised, and when used to satisfy each of the nine laws each day, will bring you fitness and good health, as surely as the sun will rise tomorrow morning.

The obvious question becomes, is practising these fundamentals each day not too hard to do? I previously mentioned the first step is desire. If we continue to do what we have always done, we are certain to get the results we currently experience. For us to get a more desirable result, we may need to tweak and change a few things. We can be sure that change is inevitable – we are either getting healthier or getting sicker, growing stronger or becoming weaker, having more energy or are tired more of the time, becoming wealthier or going in the other direction. Nature provides the evidence that nothing stays the same. Everything has an ebb and flow – the tides, seasons, and weather are constantly changing, and so can our health.

You have picked up this book for a reason. You want excellent lifelong health or are already healthy and want to stay that way. If some changes are what you need, you are now on the road to making those changes, so you can successfully realise your health goal.

This book presents the nine laws clearly. They are simple prerequisites that bring excellent health, vitality, abundant energy, mental and physical fitness, and the possibility of a long, healthy life. By applying these nine laws each day, you will find that you grow healthier, fitter, smarter and feel younger.

> *"The ball is always in your court"*

The 9 Laws of Health

My Story

I spend my early childhood years in the suburbs of Sydney, where I was plagued with illness. I suffered with respiratory problems and for as long as I can remember, I was in and out of hospital with Asthma and Bronchitis. I recall gasping for air at my bedroom window many nights, trying to breathe, only to find my gasping for air waking my brother and parents. I would end up being whisked off to hospital to spend the next few days on a drip, being filled with penicillin to get rid of the bacteria in my lungs, Ventolin to open my airways, and various other drugs to prevent me from having asthma attacks. You could be forgiven if you described me as a weak and sickly child, unable to play sports because I would wheeze and end up having an asthma attack.

I was fortunate that my diet while I was a young boy was excellent, as my father was a successful restauranteur. Dad would bring home fantastic, cooked dishes from the restaurant – freshly crumbed veal, rump or T-bone steak were favourites. He would marinate then roast chicken and vegetables. We had lots of fresh fruit and salad, and of course yummy Greek food. He would not allow us to eat foods like sausages, Chiko rolls, and the myriad of greasy options often found in take away shops. We never ate McDonald's, or Kentucky Fried Chicken and Coca Cola was forbidden.

I guess as a child I took the good family life and abundance of healthy food for granted and did not pay much attention to how well we were being looked after as children.

As I grew older, I left home at sixteen. My asthma was still with me, however, doctors said I was a lot better and I would likely grow out of it, as long as I did not start smoking. As many kids are in their early teens, I was offered a cigarette, being told it is cool to smoke.

Of course, I tried it and then I wondered what all the fuss was about! This was terrible, tasted disgusting and made me cough. I could hear my doctor and parents saying if you smoke with Asthma you will not have a very good or long life like your Greek relatives. Well, that was it – I never started smoking.

Despite all the doctor visits and good food while I was young, I did not really have a clue how to look after my own health. When I would eat, I would choose hamburgers, fish & chips, and meat pies, and wash it down with a large bottle of soft drink. I still did not eat sausages; I was turned off sausages when I saw them being made at the butcher shop owned by my school friend's father.

I did try a German sausage and found this kind of sausage to be delicious, so I became hooked. In October each year, the annual Oktoberfest was held in the city. When this time came around, a group of friends and I would venture into the city, drink large quantities of German beer and of course, eat a few German sausages.

This habit of drinking beer and eating large quantities of food continued into my twenties. On one occasion, I recall joining with friends at Pizza Hut to see how much pizza we could consume. I took out first prize by eating one and a half family sized pizzas (24 large slices) in that sitting. It did not make me sick; I was pretty full and otherwise not fazed by the experience.

I did not put on much weight, despite not being all that sporty. I did enjoy a surf when I could get to the beach between work, TAFE studies, parties, and clubbing. I love live music; so, as the years passed, I did less surfing and more partying.

In June 1988, I embarked on an adventure of a lifetime, when I applied for a job advertised in the Sydney Morning Herald. The ad read "Australian Safari - no experience necessary, all training provided, all travel and accommodation expenses provided." I thought, "WOW, this is too good to be true, I had better go for it." To cut a long story short, I ended up in Perth, Western Australia selling encyclopaedias, and loved it.

I found myself as a travelling salesperson in a team of English, New Zealand, American, Canadian, and European backpackers visiting every corner of Australia, from the tiniest towns with a general store, pub and not much else through mining towns and then onto capital cities. This lifestyle was filled predominantly with unhealthy habits, fast food, alcohol, and no exercise, apart from the odd hike into a beautiful tourist spot or lookout. If this sounds like you, brace yourself; it is going to get ugly before it gets better.

It took about three years to destroy my health and become riddled with disease. I ended up with an infected lymphatic system, septicaemia, and bowel cancer. Let me go back about a year when things started to go wrong. In July 1990, sores appeared on my arms legs and face. Despite visits to various GP's and casualty departments of two hospitals, my treatment consisted of acne cream followed by a cortisone cream, them back to the acne cream. I had a Basel Cell Carcinoma (BCC) removed from my chest in Cairns Base Hospital in January 1991. The creams did heal the various skin sores temporarily, only to have them pop up on another part of my arm or leg. They just would not go away and continued to get worse during 1991.

Our sales crew arrived in Mount Isa in May 1991. I was in my twenties and this is when I experienced my real life-threatening health challenge. I became too sick to even eat. Joanne had prepared chicken and salad rolls for lunch, a healthy change, something I would usually enjoy. When I refused to eat the roll, my work colleges became worried and took me to a local doctor. Fortunately for me, the treating physician who I'll call Adam, was a general practicing Doctor of Medicine, a Naturopath and Iridologist; as well as an Alternative Health Practitioner, trained in Traditional Chinese Medicine and Homeopathy. I really did not understand any of that stuff at the time.

I was sick and felt terrible. When Adam looked at me, I could see the concern on his face. He examined my skin, nails, and hair. He then took my right hand and then my left, to obtain pulses on each wrist – apparently each wrist corresponds to nine organs. He said he could tell the health of specific organs by the pulse at various positions and depth on each wrist. Then Adam examined my eyes, as he wanted to confirm the markings on my iris corresponded to organ disease that he felt while checking my pulses.

He diagnosed my poor state of health for what seemed like hours; however, it was just over forty minutes. This was the longest time I could ever remember being seen by a doctor. I was used to the five-minute consultation and a prescription, then being sent on my way.

Although Adam was thorough in his examination, I thought he was nuts, until he proceeded to describe where I was feeling pain in my body. He said, "Your liver is failing, your kidneys are infected, you have severe pain in your groin on both sides and under each arm pit, you bleed when you pass your stool." Nowadays with 'PC' they say, 'open your bowel' He was spot on. Adam said, "I want to take a blood and stool sample, as I believe you have septicaemia and I'd like to rule out early signs of bowel cancer."

Adam then took some blood, a stool sample, ran a few tests, he prescribed some little white pills, that looked a bit like those fake sugar substitute pills. He said it was a Homeopathic remedy that would help me relax, then insisted on bed rest until the blood test results came back, and to come back to see him in two days. It felt like I was deteriorating at an alarming rate. I still had the sores on my arms and legs and was putting this cream on that made the sores only partially heal, only to reappear worse on skin nearby.

On my next visit to the doctor, he confirmed I had septicaemia with systemic organ failure imminent and I had polyps growing in my bowel that was causing me to bleed when I opened my bowel. He said this is the early stages of bowel cancer. I must admit I had noticed blood on the toilet paper for quite a while before this time, but there was no pain going to the toilet, so I thought it must be from something I had eaten.

He said to me, "If you don't change what you are doing, that is your lifestyle, you are going to die at a very young age." This came as a shock to me. I knew I was ill, but the cancer word – going to die – was Adam for real?!

It turns out he was fair dinkum. He then said; You have three options: You can go into hospital to have the polyps removed with any cancerous large intestine, then you can have radiation therapy, but I'm concerned your blood is so toxic you may not survive the surgery; or you can carry on as you are and you will probably die; or I can treat you using an alternative therapy. I immediately thought whatever alternative therapy was, it had to be better than dying or getting my bowel cut out and having to carry around and then empty a poo bag for the rest of my life.

He then said, "Do you really want to live?" To which I replied, "Of course I do." He then offered me an alternative that included a very strict diet and lifestyle change. I thought to myself, was I ready for this? When presented with the option of dying, YES, I was ready to try anything.

The diet consisted of raw juices, any juice as long as it was raw, nothing pasteurised. You might ask as I did, Why? Adam said cooked food stops the rapid detox and increases the risk of the cancer getting out of control. Adam warned me that after a few days I would feel sicker than I currently did, and if I were worried, to come back to see him. I went back again to see Adam after 3 days, he examined me again and reassured me to continue the raw juice. It was then that he warned me I may find my body and sores will weep more as I started to cleanse.

I continued on the raw juice diet and within 2 weeks I was so ill I became bed ridden. Adam assured me to continue. I had lost 15kg but looked and felt terrible. The sores over my body were weeping badly, then I lost my big toenail. When my big toenail fell off my toe tip became an outlet for toxins. I found each morning I had to peel the sheets off my foot as they were soaked with a puss-like substance. I was so weak I was only able to walk short distances and drink the raw juices.

When I returned to see Adam again, I had been following the strict diet regime for a month. He was very pleased with this result, commenting the severe cleansing may continue for a number of weeks, then the sores would heal and disappear.

After about two months I could not take the cleansing anymore. I called Adam, who then recommended that I start eating raw foods, but I should continue with the juices as well; however, no roasted nuts, nothing cooked, not even a cup of tea. I was also advised to drink at least two litres of clean water every day with a pinch of unrefined sea salt added to some of the water I was drinking. He insisted that if I wanted to heal my body completely, I would need to maintain a raw diet for at least seven to nine months, to allow all my soft body tissue, cells, and organs to be repaired and replaced. Adam also recommended that should I then choose to eat cooked food; I should maintain a vegetarian diet.

The severe cleansing reduced over the next two weeks, and many of the sores had healed, except for my big toe that continued to weep at a reduced rate. I was eating as many different coloured fruit and vegetables as I could find, as this gave me the variety I needed. Raw nuts, honey and cold pressed olive oil were then introduced to satisfy my hunger that had now completely returned.

After three months had passed, all the sores had healed, my strength was returning and my toenail was beginning to grow back, albeit in two pieces on a slight angle. I was able to walk and go back to work and resume a normal life. I maintained the raw diet for seven months, where my complete recovery was nothing short of a miracle. I had no pain anywhere in my body and felt fantastic.

I felt this was a good time to introduce cooked foods again to my diet. I began with rice and steamed spinach, with the rest of my food still being raw. Slowly I introduced more flavour, with herbs and spices in my cooked foods and small amounts of cheese and eggs; however, I maintained a vegetarian diet for over two years.

My life was completely changed by this experience and I was on a quest to understand human health and how lifestyle habits and our environment contribute to our wellbeing, or the lack of it. I devoured every book I could find on health and diet and attended every health seminar I could find.

I joined the Natural Health Society in 1992 and in 1993 I attended the World Congress on Cancer that was held in Sydney. Speakers from around the globe presented their views on cancer and its causes, with the common theme that appeared to run through the conference that all cancer, except for possibly leukaemia, was preventable and curable, provided the conditions of the body were arranged so that the body could heal itself. This was a huge claim; however, after my experience, I do not believe we can cure cancer with a pill; rather, we should give the body what it needs to maintain excellent health and the then let the body heal itself.

From my personal experience and hearing the speakers at the conference, I was convinced at that time that cancer would be a thing of the past within a very short time, certainly by the year 2000. As everyone who reads this book probably knows, cancer has increased at an exponential rate since that time. Why? Possibly because there is no profit to be made in cancer being cured, especially if it is the body that is doing the healing.

The really big profits come from treating cancer and doing the research for a cure. Anyone who has observed the funding merry-go-round pertaining to research for a cancer cure will recall statements like, 'Cancer cure is on the horizon' or 'Human trials of a new cancer drug are just around the corner' or 'Scientists have discovered the genes that cause cancer.' It is interesting to note these statements are made right about when government funding for cancer research is about to dry up. It is unlikely a 'cure' for cancer will be found in our lifetimes by pharmaceutical companies or the cancer research institutes and foundations, for the reason stated above.

In 1998 I returned to full time studies, to further satisfy my ongoing quest to understand environmental influences and impacts on human health. I enrolled in the Public Health Science degree, selecting a major in Environmental Health. I believed this study would provide the essential understanding of body chemistry, physics, anatomy, physiology, microbiology, and life sciences to help me on my way.

I learnt a great deal about the human body and environmental influences on health at university; however, found the degree was designed to create Environmental Health Officers for local and state government jobs. As a result, I spent the next fifteen years in local government in various environmental health related roles, and a number of short deployments in developing countries to provide environmental health services.

Further studying of the brain revealed the psychological influences, including motivational forces and personal development material that can impact, and to some extent determine drivers of human thought – why we do and say what we do, and how the human thought process impacts wellbeing and healing.

Environmental factors as diverse as social interrelations, belief systems and external natural environmental factors, body physiology, physical exercise, rest, chemical and biological toxins, are all collectively impacting our internal environment. These factors in isolation are able to influence human health and wellbeing. However, when examined collectively, it becomes apparent that an absence of one determinant of health leads to disease. These discoveries have led me to understand that there are nine laws that are prerequisites of health and wellbeing.

This book has 3 distinct parts

1. The external natural environment health influences
2. The biological influences for the physical body
3. The psychological influences of the subconscious mind

Each distinct part contains three of the nine laws that are all prerequisites for health. The nine prerequisites are interdependent, as are the systems found in nature, and as found in the human body.

The Natural Environment Health Influences

Sometimes it can be challenging to satisfy this part; however, the importance of our external natural environment cannot be understated. Put simply, we all need sunshine, clean air and clean water. The mechanism to attain these prerequisites and the reasoning is explained further in the chapter on the external natural environment.

The Biological Influences of the Physical Body

Our body requires rest, exercise, and wholesome foods so that when combined with the elements of the external natural environment, and bio cybernetic psychological influences that contribute to biological processes, we ensure that chemical balance is possible. This section is explained in the chapter on the physical body.

The Influences of the Subconscious Mind

This is the most important part. Our minds need a purpose, positive loving relationships, and a sound belief system. This is so our brain can direct the body to satisfy the natural environmental health influences and obtain and satisfy the biological needs of the physical body for the benefit of the whole.

When the biological and external natural environmental prerequisites are being met, the mind has the capacity to direct the brain to effectively control all functions of the body. This can create a 'catch twenty-two': for example, the mind can choose to ignore any of the inputs through the five senses – see, hear, smell, taste, and touch – and therefore the importance of the external natural environment, or the biological needs of the physical body, thereby compromising the mind's ability to satisfy the psychological prerequisites.

When a person has grown up where some or all the elements above were not being satisfied, the subconscious mind will likely conflict with this information and the new routines desired by the conscious mind. Old habits tend to routinely surface as they have in the past. This could cause you to reject the new information, which would be an error. The chapter on the mind explains why in detail, providing an understanding of the correct use of the mind.

You can observe as I and thousands of others have – where there is a definite absence of any one of the nine prerequisites for health, or an ignorance of the laws behind the nine prerequisites for health, disease manifests within the body systems. Disease occurs when systemic interdependence between the mind and body systems loses balance. Simply explained, all the systems that control the day-to-day functions in the human body are related to one another, and a failure of one system may severely impact the functions of another system. For example, the circulatory system pumps blood from your heart throughout your body, relies on the lungs to oxygenate the blood so it can carry oxygen and further relies on the digestive system to extract the nutrients from our food to be carried in the blood to the trillions of cells and all the organs of the body.

Rather than a focus on imbalances, or disease, let your mind focus on satisfying the nine prerequisites for health daily. This daily conscious awareness will eventually be planted into your subconscious mind, where habits will be formed that will ensure the ongoing success of your health goals.

As you read this book, each of the nine laws of health are explained simply and serve as a reminder and quick reference at a later date. Read this book often until the habit of satisfying these prerequisites for health are implanted deep in your subconscious, then living and applying the nine laws will become habitually lived on a daily basis.

Part 1 – Environmental Influences

Part 1 – Environmental Influences

The external natural environment health influences are such an important component to human wellbeing that it requires a closer look. When we think of the environment, we generally think of nature. This is good because nature was the first environment. Humans have modified the living environment with technology and expertise to create a built environment that provides all the comforts we have become accustomed to. This unfortunately has come at a price. Our water is no longer H_2O with essential minerals; it is more like H_2O with a mixture of toxic water treatment and disinfection products. Read on, there is hope. Our indoor air is polluted with plastics releasing toxic gases, and often outdoor air is polluted with vehicle and industrial emissions. Read on, there is hope. Luckily, the sun rises every day; do we get enough? Our body relies on a supply of clean water, fresh air, and sunshine.

Clean Air

Why is the air we breathe so important?

Our bodies require a constant supply of oxygen to maintain all the vital systems for life. The brain, nervous, metabolic, and circulatory systems require a constant flow of oxygen being delivered to them via the lungs. Polluted air contains a multitude of contaminants that add a burden to our systems. These contaminants need to be managed and effectively eliminated from the body to maintain wellness.

Clean air is a prerequisite for good health, longevity, and overall wellbeing. Look for opportunities to get amongst living vegetation, go to parks with lots of trees, walk when the traffic stops at night. If you are in the city, well, sometimes traffic does not stop, so you will need to find some parks and nature.

How do we breathe for optimum health?

Deep abdominal breathing is not only important; it is vital to ensure the blood remains highly oxygenated. My personal research has led me to the conclusion that several deep abdominal breaths of clean air, multiple times each day, will ensure the body is able to utilise the oxygen brought in through the lungs most effectively, to cleanse the unwanted matter from the body at a cellular level.

Our lungs have the potential to store up to three litres of air, and during vigorous exercise over four litres. At rest we barely use one litre of our lung volume. This explains why many run out of breath faster than they should.

A term you may be familiar with is abdominal breathing, which is just effective deep breathing. Effective deep breathing is best achieved by standing comfortably outside, preferably where there are trees and minimal pollution from vehicles and industry. Take a full deep breath in through the nose for a count of three, draw the air down into your lungs until you feel your abdomen expand. Hold the breath for a count of nine, then exhale for a count of six out through your mouth. Research suggests that the ratio of 1:3:2 or breathe in three seconds: hold nine seconds: breathe out six seconds is the most effective to rapidly oxygenate the blood and aid the elimination of toxins.

To increase the lung holding capacity, you can, while breathing in, raise your arms in front of you then up over your head as you inhale, then back down to your side while holding and exhaling. Try to remain relaxed while doing the deep breathing. Do ten breaths at least, preferably two to three times each day. As a minimum, do at least ten breaths in the evening before going to bed, which will ensure a deep and restful sleep.

As you inhale, let the breath become so full that you experience an expansion throughout the entire abdomen area and chest cavity, feel your body fill with clean air, enjoy knowing that your lung capacity is being increased, your blood is being oxygenated and toxins are being removed from your body. Smile and know this is doing you good.

You cannot over inhale. When your lungs fill to capacity, the body will automatically begin to exhale as a result of oxygenation. Holding this breath helps develop the alignment elements of the body and provides a means of maintaining the structural integrity of the body. Over time the normal breathing capacity or tidal volume of the lungs will increase, allowing more time of vigorous exercise before running out of breath.

What is in the air we breathe?

The air we breathe is made up of mostly nitrogen, oxygen, and carbon dioxide, with traces of other gases. The quantity and type of other gases determines the quality of the air.

Normal clean air is made up of:

79% Nitrogen
20% Oxygen
1% Carbon Dioxide

How does air pollution affect our health?

Particles within aerosols may deposit themselves in different parts of the respiratory tract, depending upon their size and shape. Particles greater than ten microns (one hundredth of a millimetre) are caught in the nasal passages. These larger particles account for the production of nasal mucus (snot). The level of airborne pollutants and level of general health determine the production and composition of snot.

As particle size drops, the further the particles can go into the body and blood stream. A particle of around five microns will lodge in the larger branches of the respiratory tract. These smaller particles account for the production of phlegm. The type of airborne pollutants and level of general health determine the production and composition of phlegm.

If the particle size drops to 2.5 microns or less, they will likely travel to the alveoli of the lungs. When these small particles – I will call them absorbed contaminants – travel to the alveoli, they may also enter the blood stream. Depending on the nature of the contaminant, it may cause an infectious disease or poisoning within the body. Certain criteria determine the effect of the contaminant.

Viability – Does the body's environment support continued life of the contaminant? The body has an amazing capacity to kill or quarantine certain contaminants and effectively eliminate them from the body before they do any damage.

Concentration – Is the concentration of the contaminant high enough to be considered an infective dose or toxic dose? A diluted contaminant into the air will be further diluted as it travels in the open air.

Persistence – How long will the contaminant remain suspended in the air so that it can be inhaled? Small particles can easily be transported through ventilation systems.

Distance – What is the distance from the source of the contamination? Generally smaller particles will travel further and remain in the environment for longer.

Time – How long is the exposure to the contaminant? Spending long periods of time exposed to contaminants occurs generally when the contaminant is present where you sleep or work.

Organic – Will the contaminant mix with other chemicals in the body? Volatile Organic Compounds (VOC) are contaminants that may dissolve and become soluble and specifically interact with body fluids. Inorganic chemicals cause an immune response, where the body systems try to capture the contaminant and transport it out of the body. Sometimes inorganic contaminants cannot be eliminated and can manifest in disease later in life. The classic examples are asbestos fibres and heavy metal accumulation.

Susceptibility – How robust is the immune system of the person exposed? These factors are influenced by age, general health, chronic illness and amounts and types of medications being taken.

It is important to control air quality to maintain good health. This can be best achieved with good cross ventilation where the air quality outside is good. Where air quality is generally poor outside, good quality ventilation and filtration is the best solution. A selection of indoor plants will help to oxygenate recirculated air. It is important to note that recirculated air without plants or air exchange with the outside will result in elevated levels of carbon dioxide. High levels of carbon dioxide will induce tiredness and eventual asphyxiation.

When driving your car in the city, you generally have the ventilation in the car set to recirculate. Fortunately, car manufacturers have designed the recirculate setting to allow a small amount of outside air to enter the car while it is moving. This prevents the carbon dioxide level increasing to a dangerous level. If the car is not moving, you need to access some outside air by opening the window or setting the ventilation to outside air with the fan on.

Alternative breathing techniques.

- Get comfortable in bed or on a comfortable reclining lounge in an area with good clean air and cross ventilation. Put your arms by your side and legs out in a relaxed comfortable position. You might want to put a pillow under your knees.
- Close your eyes and listen to your breath, visualise the air entering and leaving your body.
- Breathe in deeply through your nose and out through the mouth for 5 long, even breaths.
- Inhale through your mouth and feel the air go down your throat into your lungs and back out again through your mouth, feel the breath move in and out.
- Take a deep breath in and hold it for as long as is comfortable.

Think of a dog panting, create the image of a panting dog while you are breathing in, concentrate on the inhalation, breathing in as deeply as you can, keeping the body full of oxygen; only exhale as you must, because you are so full of oxygen. Feel your rib cage expand up with a full deep breath, expanding to the stomach and lower back. Relax your arms, hands, legs, and feet, feel your body float with oxygen flowing through your body.

- When you exhale, only allow half the breath to flow out through your mouth from the abdomen.
- Hold the air in the chest, and if any of the air in the chest escapes, breathe more in.

- Continue to inhale and exhale half the breath slowly through your mouth.
- Repeat this breathing as you maintain the structural alignment of your whole body.
- Put your hands on your chest and stomach until you are comfortable and confident your body has accepted the pattern of half breathing and is holding the air in your lungs.
- As your mouth becomes dry, alternate to your nose until you are able to move back to your mouth.
- You may like to do this breathing technique for ten to fifteen minutes or as long as is comfortably possible.

If you feel any slight trembling in your upper body, your breath is travelling deeper into your body into areas where your muscles previously restricted this; this is a good sign of oxygenation, nothing to be concerned about.

- Slow down your breathing as you feel the breath move in and out of your body.
- Trust your body's natural intelligence and continue only if you are comfortable to do so.

After a while you may experience tingling in your arms and head. Eventually this will travel throughout your body and down your legs. This is good, you are oxygenating your body and this is quite normal.

When you get up and resume your normal routine you may feel taller and lighter. Experiment with these alternative breathing techniques to find the one that suits you best. The most important part is that you practise some deep breathing each day.

Plants that clean your air environment.

There has been some excellent research into plants that assist with air cleansing in polluted environments.

- Areca Palm – used by NASA in space program
- Money plant – removes formaldehyde and other VOC's, reduces eye irritation, headaches, and respiratory illness. Put two plants per 3m x 3m room where VOC's are present
- Mother-in-law's tongue – in your bedroom for max CO2 to O2 if you have your windows closed at night – six to eight waist height plants per person.

Clean water

Why is clean water so important?

Water is a natural diuretic. When our water consumption increases, we should do it gradually in line with urine production. When our urine production increases, we can increase our water intake. When we urinate, we lose salts; so, it is a balance as the salts must be replaced.

Salt can increase water retention, particularly when we are inactive. If suffering from oedema, salt should be restricted for a few days while water intake is increased, and the body is brought back to balance, then unrefined sea salt needs to be included in the diet.

When the body is well hydrated, blood volume expands, ensuring oxygen and immune system support cells can be transported effectively throughout all the tissue of the body. Blood is about 94% water; cells are about 75% water. Water osmotically enters cells and helps cells manufacture energy, so they perform optimally, and therefore are more able to excrete their waste back into the blood stream for elimination.

To quote the Iranian Doctor Freydoon Batmanghelidj, who pioneered much of the research into the importance of hydration:

99

> *"You are not sick, you are thirsty.*
> *Don't treat thirst with medication."*

There is now evidence that supports dehydration to be a contributory factor in degenerative diseases, lupus, multiple sclerosis, cancer, obesity, depression, hypertension, angina, arthritis, asthma, and adult onset of diabetes. A state of dehydration most certainly will cause pain in the body that will often manifest as headaches, muscular pain, and peptic ulcers.

When the fluid around the brain is reduced, the brain becomes dehydrated and starts to hurt. The brain requires regular flushing with clean water to remove mucus. The mucus build-up inhibits the brain's ability to effectively switch electrical impulses, resulting in lack of clarity, poor decision making and poor memory. As a minimum, it takes 500ml of water, three times per day, just to look after brain function.

How much water do we need to drink each day?

As a guide, you should drink at least 30 ml of water for every one kg of body weight. For example, an 80 kg person would drink 2.4 litres of water per day: more in hotter weather or when exercising.

Drink two glasses of water when you wake up in the morning. It is also good practice to add 5ml of quality apple cider vinegar, or lemon juice to your first glass of water in the morning. During the day, particularly in hot weather, add a gram of sea salt to a litre water bottle, and some honey to make a delicious electrolyte drink. You will benefit from increasing the daily sea salt intake in hot weather and when doing extra exercise. Drink some water a few hours before going to bed in the evening.

Should we drink with or before meals?

Yes, it is good to drink water before a meal, as the water will be absorbed by the body and secreted into the stomach in preparation to assist with digestion of solid foods. If you are thirsty during a meal, drink water. Our bodies are designed to digest water-rich foods and it is a myth that drinking water before or during a meal will disrupt digestion. Dehydration during or as a result of a meal is definitely something to avoid.

A little bit about Salt

We need at least three grams of sea salt every day. Table salt does not count and is actually bad for you, as it is not a balanced salt. Table salt is stripped of the essential trace elements. Table salt contains sodium, chloride, anticaking agent and sometimes iodine and nothing else. The major constituents of sea salt are ions Sodium, Chloride, Sulphate, Bicarbonate, Magnesium, Calcium, Potassium, Bromide, Borate, Carbonate and Strontium. There are many other trace elements and minerals essential for health that are found in sea salt. In table salt, these have been stripped out in the refining process, to be sold as elements for manufacturing processes in industry. A little sea salt in water with a ratio of 1g per litre is good in hot weather, when we are active. Sea salt is also great on food, and salt is a natural flavour enhancer.

If you find the adding of sea salt causes you to put on weight, drink more water without salt for a couple of days and your body will pass the excess fluid. You will learn what the right amount of sea salt is for your body to maintain balance, as you observe your body's response to salt consumption.

Rock salt is also good in moderation; however, sea salt is far superior. Many of the rock salts mined around the planet contain significant amounts of heavy metals that are not good for the body, such as lead, mercury, and cadmium. Aluminium is also present in significant amounts.

Benefits of Sea Salt.

- Contains many essential trace minerals required by the body,
- Regulates the water content of the body,
- Natural antihistamine,
- Anti-stressor of the body,
- Removes acidity from within cells, kidneys, and the brain,
- Improves emotional balance, and reduces depression,
- Preserves serotonin and melatonin level in the brain,
- Essential amino acids tryptophan (used to make serotonin, melatonin, indolamine, and tryptamine) and tyrosine are not used up as chemical antioxidants when sufficient water and sea salt is present in the body,
- Stabilises heart rate and blood pressure,
- Stabilises respiration,
- Removes mucus and phlegm from the lungs,
- Stabilises blood sugar levels,
- Increases electrical energy, power generation within cells,
- Improves nerve cells and information processing,
- Improves electrical energy transfer within the brain,
- Increases nutrient absorption in the gastrointestinal tract,
- Reduces tendency to cramp,
- Reduces arthritic pain,
- Strengthens bone tissue,
- Improves libido to maintain sexuality,
- Assists efficiency of venous and lymphatic system,
- Maintains muscle tone and strength,

Unrefined sea salt helps maintain electrolyte and osmotic balance. It also has an alkalizing effect on the body; the mineral content is how drinking water achieves alkalinity. Natural unrefined sea salt contains more than twenty other trace elements and minerals that the human body needs to be healthy.

The unbalanced mineral content of table salt causes mineral imbalances, being 99% sodium chloride, void of calcium and magnesium, which are two vital minerals that to a degree are available in unrefined sea salt.

If mineral depletion is not bad enough, common table salt often has aluminium. This is a toxic metal in excess, when added as a flowing agent. Table salt is often bleached for whiteness with other toxic chemicals. It is an unbalanced, toxic product that should be totally avoided.

Industry heats sea salt to boil off all the minerals, leaving virtually pure sodium chloride, then maybe adding a bit of anticaking agent, and if you are lucky a bit of potassium iodide. Pharma then repackage some of those wonderful elements and minerals that industry removed, and then they resell them back to you as mineral supplements to supplement the damage caused by the overconsumption of refined foods void of essential vitamins and minerals.

Common table salt is so refined, making it one of the worst junk foods, especially when combined with refined sugary drinks, refined foods and trans fats – more on that in the food section. Oh, you will find plenty of credentialed professionals telling you table salt and sea salt are no different from each other. Some will even tell you table salt is better when it has added iodine. Natural sources of iodine are sea vegetables, seafood, dairy products, eggs, and you guessed it, sea salt.

Sunshine

How important is sunlight in your life?

The light from the sun gives life to every living thing on our planet's surface, including our bodies.

Sound scientific evidence suggests morning sunlight and late afternoon sunlight is best for three reasons.

- Firstly, the sun is lower in the sky and therefore less intense. When the sun is at its hottest during the day the sunlight can deplete the body of energy.
- Secondly, you can spend more time in the sun around sunrise and sunset without burning and causing premature skin damage.
- Thirdly, we can all recall a time when we had the privilege to witness a spectacular sunrise or sunset. The more of these majestic displays you see, the better effect this will have on your mental health and your feelings of wellbeing.

There is new research that says you need to get out in the sun when it is near its zenith. I do not need to go into who funds this research, except to say, think about it. There is also research that says staying out in the midday sun for more than ten minutes will result in skin damage, depending on your skin type.

What does sunshine do in your body?

Photons from the sunlight cause important chemical reactions on our skin and bodies and they react with essential fatty acids like omega 3 and omega 6. Our bodies need sunlight for mental health and to produce vitamin D. Sunlight provides the natural source of vitamin D through the synthesis of cholecalciferol, from cholesterol found on the skin. Vitamin D is important for Calcium and

Phosphorus absorption, and small amounts are also found in some foods. More on that in the wholesome food section.

Johanna Budwig was a respected scientist and a PhD biochemist, who lived well into her nineties, only to pass on as a result of a fall. Budwig lived with good health and did some excellent work on the effects of sunlight – protons and the interrelationship body electrons and fatty acids have on maintaining good health.

Over time, life is depleted from all living things, without exposure to sunlight. The question that stands to follow: how much sunlight do we need, and when is the best time to get it?

The scientific evidence and my research suggest that twenty to thirty minutes enjoying a sunrise or sunset combined with deep breathing and light exercise is sufficient to maintain the sunshine prerequisite for health and wellbeing.

If you are able to enjoy both sunrise and sunset, all the better for you.

Before we move onto the physical and biological aspects of the health prerequisites, I want to touch on the social environment we were raised in. This cannot be underestimated as a controlling force where many of our beliefs, habits and paradigms were formed. We may have beliefs about our environment that could cause us to reject the importance of clean air, water, and sunshine. If this is you, read on to the section about the mind.

Part 2 – Biological and Physical Body

Part 2 – Biological and Physical Body

Each day is generally filled with important things to do and places to be. However, to satisfy the laws of the biological systems within the physical body, we need to set aside enough time to do this.

Research suggests that a reliable analysis of the needs of the human body that has passed puberty, is that ten hours out of every twenty-four hours should be set aside for rest, exercise and eating wholesome foods. Some teenagers actually need more than ten hours each day. Ok, I can hear some of you saying, "No way! You have got to be kidding! There is no way I can do this." Yes, you can, and I am going to show you how in this part of the book. We will call these biological and physical laws self-care.

Sleep, Rest and Meditation

What is it about sleep that makes it so important?

Sleep allows the body to slow down the autonomic nervous system. What is the autonomic nervous system? This is the part of the nervous system of the body that is primarily looked after by the subconscious and to a large extent, its functions are out of our control. Some of these functions include respiration, the heartbeat, and the digestive system.

There are two parts to the autonomic nervous system. Firstly, the parasympathetic nervous system is our resting and digesting phase. This is vital to maintain balance and wellbeing. The other part of the autonomic nervous system is the sympathetic nervous system, which gives us our fight and flight response. Sleep, rest, and meditation all help our autonomic nervous system get back into balance and allow our subconscious and conscious mind to sort out and file all the stimuli from our waking state.

Much of the sound research suggests the average person over eighteen years old requires seven to eight hours' sleep per night. Younger children require more – school age children require eight to eleven hours' sleep each night, preschool children require eleven to thirteen hours' sleep each day and babies up to seventeen hours' sleep each day. Although many adults appear to get by on four to six hours sleep per night, this should not be sustained.

When the body is deprived of sleep, the conscious mind becomes irrational and ill-equipped to deal with the constant flow of information coming into the brain through the five senses – see, hear, smell, taste, and touch. Part 3 of this book gets into the workings of the subconscious and conscious mind and the impact this has on brain function; therefore, I will only touch on the mind here.

The subconscious mind never sleeps and continues to gather and process information and is responsible for our dreams. The subconscious mind uses sleep time to sort through the information that has been processed by the conscious mind via the five senses during the day. When the brain is functioning properly, the conscious mind can process thousands of bits of information per second. When we awaken after a good sleep, the subconscious mind serves our conscious mind with information that aligns with our habits, beliefs and daily rituals. This is what determines which of the information coming in each second is noticed, accepted, or rejected and deleted.

Sleep deprivation inhibits the conscious mind's ability to think and sort through the information coming in, resulting in mistakes and poor judgement. A similar effect results from alcohol abuse and depressant drug use. What is actually happening in the brain? The subconscious mind is directing the brain to produce vibrations of energy, that have an amplitude and frequency. Amplitude is the maximum size or displacement of electrical energy wave from rest, and the frequency is the number of cycles from the top of each wave crest to the top of the next crest that occur in one second. The higher the vibration the more energy that is released through the body.

You might recall a friend who says they are tired all the time. What is happening when you are tired? The electrical impulses or vibrations of electrical energy generated by the brain are lower in frequency and amplitude, and the chemicals and hormones that are in exact harmony with the vibrations are also being released into the body at the same time. When we say we are tired, what we really mean is we are consciously aware that we are in a low vibration. The lower the vibration, the less effective and accurately our conscious mind is able to process the information coming in every second. We then run the risk of making conscious decisions that are not in harmony with our values and beliefs. What is even worse, the subconscious mind that controls our autonomic nervous system becomes less effective in its ability to regulate blood pressure, temperature, digestion, bladder function, and sexual function.

If this continues over an extended period, the frequency of the electrical impulses gets even lower and anxiety, fear and depression may set in. This then tends to undermine all efforts to live the laws of health. Coffee, energy drinks, some drugs and medications provide an artificial stimulus of the brain to increase electrical frequency and happy hormone production, resulting in a temporary increase of energy and vitality. Do not be fooled by this; it is an artificial stimulus that will need to be reconciled at a later time to truly enjoy vibrant health and energy. Withdrawal from these artificial stimulants can be painful, with severe headaches and erratic moods being some of the consequences.

Rest

Rest allows the body to use nutrients in the blood stream to heal and repair the body. Rest allows the filter organs of the body and the lymphatic system to accumulate waste that needs to be eliminated when the body starts to move around again. The resting metabolic rate (RMR) determines how efficient the body processes nutrients, burns fat and filters waste. This is discussed in detail in the section on exercise.

Meditation

People who regularly meditate can get by with less than eight hours sleep without a detrimental effect on their health, provided the sleep they do get is quality, and they make the time for self-care. There are many types of meditation; however, they all have one thing in common, calming the mind and focusing on a single thing (a common and easy thing to focus on is breathing). When meditating for the first time, it is difficult to focus on a single thing. Most of us at first are easily distracted by inputs from the five senses or thoughts that may brew up regarding jobs and tasks that need to be done.

Research suggests successful meditation that is gradually increased over time provides the most benefit. Initially try to calm your mind by sitting in a comfortable chair, with comfortable loose-fitting clothes, where the temperature is neither hot or cold and where you can exclude noise and inputs to your five senses. Start with a few minutes quietly feeling your breath move in and out of your body, feeling relaxed with each breath. You may want to count your breaths so you can stay focused on your breath only, allowing your mind to become stilled. To extend your meditation time, it may be helpful to run through the routine below with each part of your body while being still.

Once you have set up and are comfortable as described above and have taken ten deep breaths:

Start with your left leg, tighten the muscles in your leg from your toes to your thigh, hold for five seconds then release for five seconds,

Do the same for your right leg,

Then your buttocks and pelvic area,

Move to your left arm and tighten the muscles from your fingers to upper arm, hold for five seconds and release for five seconds,

Do the same for your right arm,

Then your shoulders,

Then your stomach,

Then your chest,

Then your back,

Then your neck.

Then your face.

Once you have done this routine you would have been going for about three and a half minutes.

If you continue with the breathing and focusing on your breath you can easily do five minutes. When you are comfortable with five minutes gradually increase this time to ten minutes.

This short, ten-minute meditation, added as part of your ten hours of daily self-care, will do so much for your mental health and feeling of wellbeing, that you will want to continue with this meditation practice every day.

Regular Exercise

Why is regular exercise so important?

Exercise done daily for thirty minutes is better than three and a half hours done once a week. Your metabolism works faster with regular exercise and your body is able to carry waste from cells through the body for elimination. Your veins don't have a pump like your arteries; they rely on muscle movement to move blood depleted of oxygen that is full of waste to be pushed through the lymphatic system and kidneys for elimination. The average person requires a combination of aerobic, strengthening and streching exercise for at least thirty minutes, three to six days per week, to maintain this prerequisite for vibrant health

What is the minimum amount of exercise we need?

Research has shown we need to do some exercise to maintain strength. Exercise allows muscles to support the skeleton and allows the body to efficiently excrete waste. Ask someone about exercise and you will likely get a different answer from every person you ask. When it comes down to it, there is a minimum amount of exercise required as a prerequisite for good health. We need a balance of stretching, aerobic and strengthening exercises to maintain bone and muscle strength and wellbeing.

The amount of exercise that is right for you will depend on your lifestyle; however, the minimum that must be done to satisfy this prerequisite for health is three times per week. Do a deliberate routine for at least thirty minutes that incorporates flexibility, strengthening and aerobic activities, every second day. Some other activity like walking or gentle stretching is beneficial on the other days.

How do we use exercise to shed weight?

If you want to shed a few or many kilograms, you will need to increase your resting metabolic rate (RMR). The easiest and most effective way to do this is doing thirty minutes of interval training that incorporates flexibility and strengthening activities, and flexibility and aerobic activities, alternating each day over six days per week. You must allow time for your body to recover; this is why you should alternate the strengthening activities and aerobic activities days. An exercise routine of seven days is not good for the body – refer to the section on rest.

Interval training is very high intensity strength or cardio activity for thirty seconds, followed by a thirty second rest period, sustained for a minimum of five minutes, to as long as thirty minutes. Prior to commencing an interval training regime, you should be able to sustain moderate cardio activity for thirty minutes without a break.

Interval training is working your body to 90% of its limits, and therefore carries significant risk if you have been living a sedentary lifestyle or only doing small amounts of exercise occasionally. Consult your doctor before starting an interval training regime and build up cardiovascular fitness over a period of time first.

Cardiovascular fitness is really the ability of your heart and lungs to supply oxygen-rich blood cells to the working muscle tissues, where they use oxygen to produce energy for sustained movement. The more efficiently your body can deliver sustained oxygen through the body, the less demand placed on your vital organs.

How long does it take to build cardiovascular fitness?

A wide body of research suggests three to four weeks; however, when you can do any of the following continuously for thirty minutes, your cardiovascular fitness should be ready for interval training.

- Power walking,
- Swimming,
- Dancing,
- Skipping rope,
- Running,
- Any high intensity sport such as soccer or basketball where you are constantly moving.

What is the resting metabolic rate?

The word metabolism is derived from Greek and means 'change' or 'transformation'. Our metabolism can be described as the sum total of all physical and chemical changes that are taking place our body. Food is digested and nutrients are adsorbed and transformed into energy, new compounds such as hormones are formed, bone and muscle tissue grow, tissues and cells are destroyed and eliminated, along with all the other body processes.

The RMR is the rate these processes continue to occur after we stop exercising, or when we are at rest or sleeping.

When we do not satisfy the biological prerequisites for health or are deficient in these biological areas, the metabolic rate decreases. Consequently, weight gain is common, and research suggests this can lead to many other health problems.

Lowering your kilojoule and fat intake is bantered around as the most important components of weight loss. This decreases your metabolic rate, so you burn fewer kilojoules, resulting in the yo-yo effect of weight loss and weight gain, with no true significant health benefits, and often causing the body to store fat reserves to account for the restricted kilojoule intake.

Our RMR can vary, depending on a number of factors; however, the most influential factors to increase the RMR are regular interval exercise, wholesome high-water content nutrient-dense food, and adequate rest.

How to get more energy?

Energy levels increase as we satisfy each prerequisite for health. However, many great traditional oriental masters have taught for thousands of years that certain deliberate movements will significantly increase the human body's energy output. Introducing Chiyotes, (pronounced chi-yo-tez), this form of exercise was developed from the teachings of the masters of Qigong, Tai Chi, Yoga and Pilates.

Chiyotes means 'way to energy' and has several distinct sets of routine movements that increase energy, flexibility, bone, muscle, and core strength.

The best thing about Chiyotes is that you can combine your strengthening core work, cardio and stretching into an easy to do and remember routine. Refer to the section on breathing and you will quickly see why Chiyotes works so well to compliment a workout and cellular cleanse. The exercises start gently and depending on your level of fitness can be as intense as you choose. Most importantly, you can complete the exercise routine in 30 minutes without gym equipment if you like.

The floor routine – five to ten minutes. This can be done in bed and is an excellent way to start your day, on an exercise mat, on the grass or on the beach at sunrise. This part of the routine also warms up the body and gets the breathing right. The floor routine done while in bed is particularly good for those with illness or injury that restricts their ability to move around.

The cleanse and core, standing routine – seven to ten minutes. This is done in the standing position, with feet generally shoulder width apart, incorporating twelve movements.

The Chiyotes standing routine aids flexibility and core strength and is described below.

You can view all the routines at <u>Wellbeing Management</u>

The cleanse and core, standing routine

For exercise one to eight, do each exercise eight times before moving onto the next one:

- Deliberately breathing from your abdomen,
- Hold each stretch for a few seconds,
- The whole routine should be done slowly and takes less than ten minutes.
- If you feel pain, back off to comfort and hold for a couple of seconds.

As you get more flexible and fitter, the exercises get much easier and you get more energy from doing them. Try to do the exercises five or six times per week.

To start, stand tall and straight with feet shoulder width apart, take three deep breaths to centre yourself before starting the first exercise.

Exercise 1 - Press the Sky – put your hands above head, with your palms facing up, feet shoulder width apart. Push upward towards sky, breathing out, hold, then lower your hands back to the starting position, repeat eight times.

Exercise 2 - Pull the Bow – breathing out, stretch one arm out to the side with your palm stretched back at right angle to outstretched arm, with the other hand form a fist close to your chest, feet shoulder width apart, turn your head in direction of outstretched arm, hold, then in a smooth motion, breathe in and swap to the other arm while breathing out, repeat four times each side.

Exercise 3 - Alternate Arm Press – your arms by your side, feet shoulder width apart, breathe out, pushing one up and other down with palm stretched back at right angle to outstretched arms, press and hold, then in a smooth motion, breathe in and swap the arms, breathing out as you press to the other side, repeat four times each side.

Exercise 4 - Spinal Rolls – standing with your head facing straight and feet shoulder width apart, breathe in, and on the outward breath roll your head forward tucking into your chin, then continue rolling down with your arm extending to the floor between your feet, hold, then roll back up breathing in as you come up, untuck your chin to return to the full standing position, repeat eight times.

Exercise 5 - Side Bends – feet shoulder width apart, breathe in, and on the outward breath stretch one arm over your head to one side in direction of the first bend, and the other arm sliding down the outside of leg towards floor, hold then breathe in as you come up and then swap sides while breathing out, repeat four times each side.

Exercise 6 - Cow Looks at the Moon – arms out in front at shoulder height with your palm stretched back at right angle to your arm, with a slight bend in your elbows, feet shoulder width apart, breathe in, on the outward breath twist your whole upper body slowly in one direction as far as you are comfortable to go, keeping arms at shoulder height and following with head, hold then breathe in as you twist back to the front starting position, then twist in the other direction as you breathe out, repeat four times each side.

Exercise 7 - Squat – feet and knees together, breathe in, and on the outward breath bring both arms back and up over your head and down in front as you go down into the squat, push your bottom out and back (make sure your knees don't go past your toes), hold, and then as you breathe in, let arms follow through behind you and up over your head as you stand up and return to the full standing position, repeat eight times.

Exercise 8 - Punches - feet shoulder width apart, breathe in, and on the outward breath with your thumbs inside a clenched fist, punch one arm fully extended forwards, fist fingers facing down, with the other arm in a clenched fist fingers facing up on your side against your ribs, hold, then breathe in, as you swap arms breathe out, repeat four times each side.

Exercise 9 - Lower Back Massage - feet shoulder width apart and rest the back of both palms on your lower back and bounce lightly on the spot letting palms lightly massage your lower back, continue for eight breaths.

Exercise 10 – Stand like a Tree – feet and knees together, then bring one leg up with the foot facing down resting on the inside of the other leg near the knee, bring both arms up over your head with your palms facing each other, stretch upward, holding your head straight, (as you get stronger you can look up at your hands) breathe deeply from your abdomen holding your core firm, work towards holding the pose for thirty breaths. Then return to the starting position and do the other leg for the same time.

Exercise 11 - Warrior Star – feet and knees together, then bring one leg out to one side with the foot at right angles to the other foot, about a one metre wide stance, lean into the outstretched leg (not allowing the knee to go past the toes) stretch both arms out at shoulder height in opposite directions. If you lead with your right leg, your right arm should be stretched in the direction of your right toes, and your head should be facing to the right, with the other arm stretched out in the opposite direction, hold your core and stance for ten breaths, then drop right arm down to the outstretched leg inside the calf muscle and the other arm stretched towards the sky, turning your head towards the sky as well, hold stance for five breaths, then repeat for the other side.

Exercise 12 - Eagle – feet and knees together, then bring one leg out in front, knee bent at waist height with the foot flat facing forward, balancing on the other leg, both arms stretched out to each side at shoulder height helps with balance, holding your core hold for three breaths, repeat two times each side.

The cardio routine – ten minutes with an interval routine, or thirty minutes sustained. The cardio routine can be done using your body or gym equipment if you prefer. The goal is to increase your heart rate to increase your cardiovascular fitness. The exercise you choose should be one you enjoy and can do at least three times per week, at least every second day.

The strengthening routine – ten minutes with an interval routine, working particular muscle groups in rotation. This can be done using your body or gym equipment if you prefer. The goal is to put a load on your muscles and bones to increase muscle strength and maintain bone density.

Warm down routine – five minutes, this is done in the standing position, incorporating two gentle movements, and breathing.

Warm down 1 – Charlie - Standing with heels together and toes pointing outward at about 45 degrees or what is comfortable for you. Knees slightly bent, arms hanging by your side, breathe in, and on the outward breath raise your heels so you are standing on your toes, legs straight and body tall. Then on the inward breath, lower your heels to the ground, returning to the start position. Repeat ten times.

Warm down 2 – Oxygenate - Standing with feet shoulder width apart with a slight bend in the knees. Hold your hands, palms facing up in front of your abdomen. Breathe in and raise your hands to your chest height, hold your breath while turning your palms outwards, pushing away from you to fully extend your arms, in a smooth motion extend your arms up over your head and down your sides as you breathe out, returning your hands to the starting position. Repeat this ten times.

Wholesome Foods

Why are wholesome foods so important to health?

Food is our fuel and our medicine, bottom line. You are what you eat. Your food provides the essential nutrients for all the other prerequisites of health. There is a great deal of controversy regarding what is good for you, what you should eat, what you should avoid. This section will cover what you need to know. Hundreds of books have been written, some are quite good, many are terrible and hundreds more could be written just on the topic of food alone. What you need are the facts, information that is logical and easy to follow, that you can apply from today. The sooner you start looking after what you put into your body the sooner you will reap the rewards that lead to perfect health.

When you become sick or overweight, it is important to realise that it takes time for your health to deteriorate. Be patient with yourself, this is a lifelong journey, it will take time to restore perfect health depending on where you are on this journey. What is important is your commitment to your goals, yourself, and your determination to succeed. You will find that applying the nine principles at some level each day you can be sure that over time, you will reach your health goal.

Fresh foods will always be superior to packet, canned and over processed foods. When shopping for food, avoid most of the aisles and head for the fresh produce, your body will thank you for it.

A bit about salts.

Salt is also essential to maintaining good health, if you have any doubt about this, consider the first thing the doctor requests when you are admitted to hospital with an injury or sickness, a saline drip. When livestock are not well a salt block is placed by their water trough. This should give you a good indication regarding the myth, 'salt is bad for you'. It is just that, a myth.

I do not consider refined salt with all the minerals removed except for sodium, chloride, and anti-caking agent as suitable salt for the body.

Sea salt or rock salt must be consumed as part of the diet to maintain electrolyte and water balance. Salt is discussed in more detail in the chapter about clean water.

A bit about diets.

Forget the fad diets! Yes, most of them will make you starve, eat food you do not like, or that when you eat it, feel like you are going to die. Between the misconceptions promoted by those with vested interests, and the speed at which the conglomerates manipulate our government regulators, to determine what is good today and bad tomorrow, how can people discern what is best for maintaining perfect health, year in, year out.

Paleo is a good example of a fad diet. The diet changes depending on who is selling the idea to you. There are many sensible food recommendations in the diet; however, the science does not support the fad elements. When one observes the contradictions such as no dairy, but butter is good, no processed meats but bacon is good, enough said.

Ketosis diet, no bread, minimal carbs lots of fats and lots of protein. The science behind this suggests that fat burning will be increased as a result of a lack of glycogen production derived from carbohydrates. While this is true in the short term, the diet is not sustainable as the body becomes acidic. When the blood stream becomes acidic, an environment for cancer cell growth is established. Cancer cells do not grow in an alkaline environment, the blood should be maintained slightly alkaline.

I have a good friend that is a little overweight who has been on this diet for over a year now. He has not lost the weight he had hoped to lose however, he does not look as healthy as he used to, and he has terrible dogs' breath. He is missing out on so many foods that we both know he enjoys eating, because he has been convinced this will help him to regain his optimum weight. He does a simple urine test to see if he is maintaining ketosis, this he does almost daily. I agreed to take the test with him to see a direct comparison. To his disbelief I was in greater ketosis than he was at the time. Personally, I would never put myself through that kind of diet.

The list goes on and on with fad diets, shakes, meal replacements; however, you do not really need any of them. Follow the nine prerequisites for health and you will attain and maintain fantastic vibrant health for the rest of your life.

It is no wonder most people feel overwhelmed and confused by all of the conflicting information and marketing regarding nutritional information. Are carbs good or bad? Is exercise the key to weight loss? Should I put butter or margarine on my toast? It's crazy, we see people bouncing from one fad diet to another, then end up going back to what they know, the habits that have been programmed into their subconscious mind over the years, back to their old, ingrained eating habits, often gaining more weight in the process.

A bit about, eat 'this' not 'that'.

We have all heard do not eat butter, margarine is best; then we hear, no, margarine is bad, butter is best. We hear a similar thing with salt; a low salt diet is best, or you will get heart disease. What about eggs; eggs are good, eggs are bad, no eggs are good, no they are bad. Meat, you need to eat red meat, no do not eat red meat, grain fed beef is best, no, grass fed is best, no, eat white meat, but do not eat pork, then get some pork on your fork, do not eat chicken it is full of hormones, no, chickens are not fed hormones, eat chicken, it is lean meat. Leave the fat on your meat, no, cut it off, no, do not cut it off, fat is good. Grains, grains are good for you, do not eat grains they are bad for you, or worse still you can only eat a certain type of grain. The marketers do not tell you it is because that grain is the one in fashion or oversupply or generates the highest profits. Please do not get me wrong, there is nothing wrong with a company making a profit; however, there is something wrong with the same company misleading people about what is good for their health for profit.

Every person is different and at different levels of health and vitality. There are multiple varieties of body types and shapes, some have allergies or intolerance to certain foods. The causes of allergies and intolerances is a whole book on its own and will not be covered here. There is evidence that many intolerances and allergies are alleviated or eliminated altogether as the body gets healthier, healing itself.

While I was growing up and in my late teens, I was always able to eat prawns; then without warning at eighteen years I developed a prawn and crustacean allergy. I would puff up around the face and hands and get rashes over any part of my body that even touched a prawn. This went on for a just over a decade. After recovering from the life-threatening illness in my twenties, I regained my health, then in my late twenties while at a friend's home I unwittingly exposed

49

myself to prawns in a fried rice dish, and to my astonishment there was no reaction to the prawn whatsoever. Over the coming months I tested prawns and other crustaceans without incident. I was cured of my allergy, and at the time I had no idea why or how this had happened.

Some of us are just born with a genetic disposition that results in poor health while we are young, and unfortunately for those of us that start with bad genes, will live a life of poor or failing health. The genetic disposition that was handed down from our parents at birth can be altered as we change our environment, that is external natural environment, social environment, internal environment, and our ruling mental state.

Research carried out by Dr Bruce Lipton, coined Epigenetics, is the study of the influence environmental factors and the ruling mental state have on every one of the billions of new cells that are created in our bodies daily. This book only touches on epigenetics in the section on the mind, however the nine laws of health explain the success of this research. New cells can mutate based on their environment and will either be better or worse depending on how we apply the nine laws of health in our lives.

What foods do we need to eat?

To keep it simple and easy to follow, we need a variety of high-water content nutrient dense foods to feed every cell in the body. The foods are made up of carbohydrates, proteins, fats, vitamins, and minerals. For those interested in the science and technical aspects of food, there is more detail in the technical section further on.

What should I be eating?

Much of the scientific evidence suggests an animal-based diet as the foundation of your meals; however, the scientific evidence also suggests this causes a decrease in overall health and increases the risk of degenerative diseases, thus reducing your lifespan. This is where you need to dig deep into who is funding the research to really know what is going on. Do not worry, you will not have to, because I have reviewed the research and put the findings to the test.

A plant based wholesome meal plan centred around unrefined foods as recommended below offer a healthy, fulfilling, and long-term solution to those that want to shed weight, gain health, fitness, and strength. Forget the yo-yo diets and binges, that amount to physical and psychological torture. Scientific evidence suggests the more plant based your meals are, the lower the kilojoule density, the leaner the protein and the better the fats. This leads to increased thermoregulation, and improved hormone balance, making it easier to satisfy all the laws of health. A simple well-balanced meal plan can be achieved using the ratio 6:2:1 of Carbohydrate: Protein: Fat, and four basic food groups that consist of mainly unrefined spray free foods:

Seeds, Nuts and Grains

Grains – millet, buckwheat, oats, brown or basmati, jasmine or long grain white rice, wheat, barley, spelt, rye, quinoa, etc.

Nuts – almonds, walnuts, pecans, macadamias, brazil nuts, cashews, pistachios, avoid peanuts unless you know they are spray free.

Seeds – alfalfa, pumpkin, sesame, fenugreek, mustard, chia, etc.

Vegetables, Beans

All vegetables, including sea vegetables; plus, beans (red kidney, mung, adzuki, lima, pinto/borlotti, butter, broad and haricot); lentils, garlic, onions, ginger, herbs, and spices.

Fruits

All fruits in season, best eaten with breakfast or between meals.

Additions

If you want to eat meat, eat it. Fish, poultry, or lean meat is best. Yoghurt, eggs, cheese, rice or nut milk, fresh unpasteurised milk (goats or cows) if these are desired.

Honey, stevia, sea salt, cold pressed oils (olive oil, grapeseed oil, coconut oil, and flaxseed oil), brewer's yeast, herbal teas, soy sauce, (Braggs or Tamari).

Remember additions are not the main part of meals.

Summary – for every handful of fat you need two handfuls of protein and six handfuls of carbohydrates, or whatever measuring container suits you. Fresh unadulterated whole foods provide vast amounts of phytochemicals. In recent decades research suggests these naturally occurring compounds found in plants, fruits, vegetables, and grains, actually assist to slow the aging process. Choose a variety fresh and high-water content, colourful foods. That way you can be sure that you get your required vitamins and minerals as well.

Processed or fresh.

We could talk a fair bit about the pros and cons of pasteurised milk products. I will say that there are good public health reasons for the pasteurisation of milk products, as intensely farmed animals may have some unwell beasts that may contaminate the milk supply before being detected and isolated from the herd. The pasteurisation ensures these milk products are safe for consumption; however, the pasteurisation process tends to make the milk acid forming in the body and the digestive enzymes contained in whole milk are destroyed. This could be a reason for some people having an intolerance for pasteurised milk.

Processed meats mostly contain preservatives that can harm your health if you eat them every day. For example, sodium nitrate and sodium benzoate are just two of the many preservatives you will be consuming too much of when you eat processed meats. These preservatives should be kept to a minimum in your food.

Processed foods are often hard to identify. Can you discern exactly what is in them? They most certainly lack what the body needs to satisfy this law of health. The most important thing is a variety of fresh high-water content, colourful foods that have had minimal processing. You may need to individualise your choice of foods according to your specific dietary and medical needs.

Whatever you do, try not to get too caught up on organic foods. In the true sense of the word, organic means derived from living matter, so faeces are organic too. The other definition for organic refers to the practice of food production without the use of artificial chemicals, pesticides, or herbicides. Unless you are absolutely sure of the organic certification body mentioned on the label, organic means nothing more than derived from living matter. Nowadays most products in the supermarket that are labelled organic, are not certified organic and are not chemical or spray free.

In some countries food is grown in human effluent and then labelled organic. I have a problem with this, as human effluent contains metabolites from the myriad of pharmaceutical medications consumed by the populations producing the effluent. There is research currently being done to determine the impact on human health and the effect on the immune system that these metabolites have. Some research suggests that these metabolites are being transferred from the effluent into the food as it grows. Consider how many women between puberty and menopause that consume the contraceptive pill, or how many people take daily medications for mental health and other degenerative disease. Need I go on?

Detoxification of the body

Should I do a General Detox?

We should all do a general detox when we feel we have been unable to satisfy any of the nine laws of health for an extended period of time. For those of us that live in large cities, our air is polluted, and our reticulated water contains a cocktail of additives used by the water authorities to clarify it, get the pH neutral and make it safe to drink.

If we are exposed through, or by ingestion, inhalation absorption through the skin or eyes to poisons, toxins, pesticides, herbicides, fungicides, or heavy metals etc, we would need to do a detox after being treated or diagnosed by a medical doctor as soon as possible after the exposure.

Foods that help to detox various organs and tissues of the body.

Arteries - Broccoli, Turmeric, Chia seeds, Oranges, pomegranate
Lymphatic System - Parsley, Myrrh, Nettle, Goldenseal, Burdock Root
Liver - Turmeric, Garlic, Beetroot, Dandelion Root
Kidney - Ginger, Apple Cider Vinegar, Lemon water
Intestines - Gooseberry, Apples, Bananas, Leek, Almonds

My grandmother gave me this recipe to detox from heavy metal contamination after the removal of my amalgam tooth fillings. 2 tablespoons (30 ml) of organic apple cider vinegar, half a teaspoon of bi-carb soda (2.5 g), mix in a glass until it stops fizzing then add a cup (250 ml) of rainwater or filtered water. Drink this for six days on then six days off for four cycles (48 days)

Please note this is not a comprehensive list, this is just a starting point. Many books have and could still be written on specific foods, herbs and formulas that will aid in detoxifying the body.

Fasting for a day is also a very good way to help detoxify the body, as it gives the cleansing organs, liver, kidneys, arteries, lymphatic system, and digestive system time without food to do a general clean up. It is very common during a sustained detox for you to become unwell for a period of time. The time and severity will vary for each person and their level of toxic load within their body prior to the detox. Always consult your doctor if you have a health condition before you do a detox or fast.

Technical information - Food

To ensure effective metabolism and available energy, the majority of foods should be alkaline forming once consumed. There is a great deal of confusion regarding acid and alkaline foods. Many acid fruits are alkaline forming when consumed. Acid and alkaline are a measure of the potential of hydrogen, abbreviated to pH. The pH scale goes from pH 1 highly acidic, through to pH 7 neutral, to pH 14 highly alkaline.

The pH of saliva first thing in the morning prior to eating or drinking should be pH 7 to 7.5 slightly alkaline. Blood should also be slightly alkaline too at pH 7.2 to 7.4 as the blood carries nutrients and oxygen throughout the body. The pH of the blood and the morning saliva pH level are often very close; however, the pH of saliva can vary if there is tooth decay or teeth were not brushed properly the evening prior to sleep. When the pH of the saliva in the morning is below pH 6.5 this is an indicator of disease within the body that needs to be addressed. You can be sure repeated saliva tests that return acidic, suggests the blood is also likely to be acidic.

Blood pH is always more stable as the blood has the capacity to buffer itself (holds the pH at a constant level). Testing the blood pH requires a visit to your doctor for a blood test. When the pH of the blood becomes acidic, this is a very serious state that needs to be addressed by a health care professional competent in dietetics and nutrition. As a result of the blood's buffering capacity, an acidic blood result may take an extended amount of time to correct.

The use of a pH test strip on the tongue first thing in the morning is the quickest and cheapest pH test and should be performed a few times each year, more often if a result ever shows a pH below 7. The testing should be done regularly until the pH balance is rectified. Alkaline forming food are an essential part of the diet to allow the body to undertake its healing processes.

The skin has an acid mantle to provide protection to the body and has a more acidic pH 4 to 5.5. This is the reason often otherwise very healthy people get skin cancers. Cancer cells thrive at pH 6.4 and below. An interesting fact about cancer is it cannot grow in an alkaline environment. Melanoma, the most serious and potentially deadly skin cancer, cannot penetrate the dermis if the blood maintains the correct pH balance.

The pH of gastric acid within the stomach pH 1.5 to 3. The body excretes juice from various organs to aid digestion before the nutrients from the digested food can be absorbed into the blood stream when they reach the small intestines.

It takes seven to nine months for your body to replace all soft tissues, such as muscles, liver, kidney, digestive tract, respiratory system, and nervous system. Your entire brain and every memory and nerve cell are replaced, every soft tissue cell of the body is replaced. Cells in the digestive tract can be replaced daily, skin cells every couple of weeks. It depends on the cells and what job they are required to perform in the body.

Before you dismiss this and say, "But I have a scar and have had it for years"; Yes, all your cells have a memory, this is referred to as cellular memory, and it works by creating the cell to replace itself from the nutrients in the blood stream in accordance with the genetic sequence for the cell's function.

The replacement cell renewal process ensures the cell is manufactured with the same composition as the cell that is being replaced, less the aging process. So, the scar is imprinted within the cell and the instruction to the new cell includes the instruction for the scar. Sometimes scars become faint over time, and this is a result of the quality of the materials being used to make the new cells. There are treatments that include tiny electrical impulses on scar tissue that can disrupt the cellular memory so that when the cell is replaced the scar disappears. Another way scars fade is the result of Level Three regeneration.

There are three levels of nutrient utilisation to run the body and they are interdependent on the other eight prerequisites for health. The priority is Level One utilisation, and only when there is sufficient surplus nutrient availability will Level Two utilisation be initiated. Most people live somewhere between Level One and Level Two nutrient availability, as a result of poor diet, misinformation, and poor lifestyle choices.

When nutrient is consumed Level One utilisation is the priority. The subconscious utilises all available resources for sympathetic and parasympathetic system function. This comprises the autonomic nervous system that can accelerate or slow the heart rate, widen bronchial passages to increase oxygen uptake, manage digestion throughout the entire digestive tract from the oesophagus through the stomach, small intestine, to the large intestine and finally the anus for elimination. The autonomic nervous system regulates blood vessel size, causes pupillary dilation or contraction, initiates goose bumps, water balances perspiration and raises or lowers blood pressure. During normal circumstances, we have little or no control over Level One utilisation. Probably the best example of our attempt to control autonomic function is when we hold our breath or hold onto a bowel movement or when we need to urinate.

Level Two utilisation is primarily concerned with repair, healing of cuts, bruising, sprains, fractures, bacterial, viral, and fungal invasions. For a normal individual with good Level Two utilisation capacity, healing is rapid. Small cuts heal completely in a matter of a few days. These people rarely get ill, when they do get exposed to bacteria or virus, their body moves rapidly to destroy invasive pathogens and they recover very quickly.

Level Three utilisation is reserved for only those who maintain a high level of nutrition, along with adherence to the other eight prerequisites over a sustained period of time. The available nutrients or raw materials at Level Three is abundant every day when all the prerequisites for health are also maintained each day. The genetic coding of cells permits superior cell formation at Level Three utilisation. The body replaces an estimated three hundred million cells every minute. The most abundant cells in the body are red blood cells which are replaced every four months. Some digestive tract cells are replaced every day while others take several months to be replaced. It is a logical consequence that when we maintain Level Three utilisation and maintain the prerequisites of health, we feel better, look younger, have more energy, life force, mental clarity, and capacity to perform at our best. We have all seen people who look well past their years, and equally we see people whose years are well past their appearance. Level Three utilisation is the reason for this phenomenon.

All cells, regardless of their location in the body, require nourishment, waste elimination and fluid balance. When a cell is in balance it is said to be healthy, as this then allows the cell to perform at its optimum genetic programming.

It takes five to seven years to replace your bones and teeth. Yes, you heard right, bones and teeth are replaced too every five to seven years. Remember everything including our bones and teeth are made up of atoms and elements. Nothing rests, when energy flows in a system that appears to be solid, like within the cells of the body's bones and teeth, the energy flow is actually movement. This movement is how the bones and teeth are being replaced; it is just happening at a slower rate, because our bones and teeth are more dense than soft tissue.

The only things in the body that are not replaced by the body are any artificial implants such as amalgam, plastic and gold fillings, pacemakers, pins, screws, and prosthetic devices. If these artificial fittings had genetic instruction encoded within the particles as cell tissues do, they too would be replaced. Research is being done to create living tissue replacement parts for the body. Time will tell how the body responds to this new technology. I expect if the body accepts the biological replacement part, it will replace the cells like any other body cells.

Calories and Kilojoules

One calorie is equal to 4.18 kilojoules.

The number of kilojoules required is dependent on the age, sex, RMR, body type and level of physical activity. For an active male who wants to maintain good health, they may consume upwards of 10,000 kilojoules per day. This can be achieved using the ratio 6:2:1 of Carbohydrate: Protein: Fat, as mentioned earlier. The active male should be getting most of the kilojoules from carbohydrates 359 grams, then protein 120 grams, then fats 53 grams. For an active woman, upwards of 7500 kilojoules per day, from carbohydrates 270 grams, then protein 90 grams, then fats 40 grams. Note, this does not include the weight of the water the body needs each day. Depending on what country you are from, the Recommended Daily Allowance (RDA) will vary considerably, and the RDA may be influenced by those that do not have your best interests at heart.

Another way to look at it is to use your current body weight or your desired body weight to determine how much food you need to maintain a particular weight. For those who are training hard or intend to compete as athletes, they may need 50% or more extra dietary intake than someone who just seeks to maintain excellent health.

For example, an endurance athlete weighing 85kg competing in a triathlon would eat plenty and need approximately the following to maintain good dietary intake.

Carbohydrates > 5.3 g per 1kg of body weight per day.
Protein > 1.8 g per 1kg of body weight per day.
Fats > 0.8 g per 1kg of body weight per day.

For a person of 85kg who wants to shed weight, the above would be way more than they really need; however, they still would need at least the following to maintain a minimum dietary intake.

Carbohydrates up to 2.7 g per 1kg of body weight per day.
Protein up to 0.9 g per 1kg of body weight per day.
Fats up to 0.4 g per 1kg of body weight per day.

To shed weight fast, however, may not be best for you so check with your doctor first. Conversely, to gain weight stay on the heavier side of the amounts for an active male or female. Remember many other contributing factors determine body weight, therefore apply this section only after studying the other prerequisites for maintaining excellent health. It is easy to get caught up in all the calorie counting, with the main problem being, when one wants to count calories, the only foods that have the nutritional information that includes calories and kilojoules are foods in packets. We do not want to be eating foods in packets most of the time, so this makes it very hard to calorie count.

Nutrients

The macronutrients are carbohydrates, proteins, and fats, and the micronutrients are vitamins and minerals. A quick and easy way to ensure the foods you eat contain sufficient nutrients, vitamins, essential fatty acids, carbohydrates, proteins, and trace minerals is to juice. I do not mean fruit juice, as fruit juice even if freshly squeezed or pressed is too concentrated in sugars. Fruit is best eaten whole, or a piece added to your vegetable juicing. 500 ml of freshly squeezed or pressed vegetable juice each day is an excellent way to help the body move to Level Three utilisation.

Drinking juices increases energy production, strengthens the immune system, glows the complexion, strengthens our organs and bones, therefore greatly increasing wellbeing. Many nutrients are bound to the fibre in fruits and vegetables, which is expelled from the body; however, we can recover more vitamins and minerals by juicing. When we juice the vegetables, their goodness is released from the fibre in the food, we are then drinking highly concentrated nutrients which enter our bloodstream very quickly.

This is not a substitute for consuming whole fruits and vegetables, which still contain essential fibre. Eating fruits and vegetables in their natural state provides us with substantial amounts of vitamins, minerals, and essential fibre. Legumes and whole grains also contain plenty of essential fibre.

Macronutrients

You could get your head into a spin sifting through the maze of carbohydrates, proteins and fats and their chemical composition, mode of action in the body, which ones to have and which to avoid; so, I am not going to get into it here. Unless you intend to be a nutritionist, keep it simple.

Carbohydrates - The basic unit of carbohydrates is a monosaccharide (glucose, fructose, galactose), disaccharide (sucrose, lactose, maltose) and polysaccharide (starch). Refined white sugar (sucrose) is the worst carbohydrate you can consume, so best kept to an absolute minimum. Carbohydrates are reduced to glucose, the simplest form through digestion, before your body can make use of them. When there is a decreased availability of carbohydrates, the body will metabolise proteins and fats to compensate as an alternative energy source.

Proteins - These are used by cells for structure. Proteins are the basis for all structural tissues' building, maintenance and repair, and therefore vital for muscle cells. Protein is vital for enzymes, antibodies, and balancing hormones within the body. Proteins are made from two or more amino acids. There are twenty different amino acids, eight of which are called essential amino acids (isoleucine, leucine, lysine, methionine, phenylalanine, threonine, tryptophan, and valine), because our body is not capable of manufacturing them.

Often some people hypothesise you cannot get all the essential amino acids if you do not eat meat; this is not true. For example, grains lack lysine but have sufficient methionine, legumes lack methionine but have plenty of lysine. A combination of grains and legumes will provide all the essential amino acids. Cooking denatures protein, therefore it is wise to get some of your daily protein from raw foods, such as nuts, seeds, and seed sprouts. Protein is also found in some fruits, such as avocado, guava, apricots, kiwifruit, and blackberries.

It is important to eat protein every day, as excess protein is not stored in the body; however, do not overdo protein consumption, as some of the fad diets suggest. Research suggests that excessive protein consumption will result in increased calcium excretion through the urine, increasing the risk of osteoporosis later in life.

Fats - These are used by cells for wall padding to protect vital organs, brain tissue and storage of energy, and act as messengers for proteins. Fats can be monounsaturated, polyunsaturated, derived mainly from plants and fish, or saturated fats mostly derived from animals, coconut, and palm oils. I do not want to get too deep into the chemistry but want to point out that polyunsaturated fat and saturated fat together should be less than 20% of our fat intake, with the remainder being monounsaturated fat. Saturated fats have the maximum number of hydrogen atoms attached to the carbon chain, resulting in a higher melting point. Saturated trans fats found in nearly all deep-fried foods are the worst fats and should be avoided.

Limit your intake of saturated animal fats, as they are solid at our body temperature. An inevitable consequence of eating foods containing animal fat at every main meal, is that the blood tends to stay fatty all day, as it takes four to five hours for the body to metabolise these types of fats. The consequence of a build-up of fatty deposits that have not been effectively metabolised is a build-up on the lining of blood vessels throughout the whole body. This in turn restricts blood supply as the lining swells, increasing blood pressure.

All the body organs that rely on an unrestricted supply of oxygen and nutrients, become starved of oxygen and are in danger of malnutrition. Further, these organs are now compromised, as the waste is no longer effectively being removed; therefore, continues to build up from cell metabolism, putrefying in an oxygen-poor environment. The inevitable result is organs function poorly and eventually fail. This is another reason such a large percentage of the population is tired, overweight, lacks energy or is afflicted with diseases. The medical term for this condition is congestive toxicosis, however this condition is reversible through simple dietary and lifestyle changes as suggested in this book.

Fats consumed in food are broken up into fatty acids, and used as above or stored as triglycerides (three fatty acid molecules, attached to a glycerol molecule), and cholesterols based on their chemistry and the needs of the body. There are also essential omega 3 and omega 6 fatty acids that the body does not produce. These essential fatty acids assist the body absorb vitamins and minerals, and most importantly, omega 3 fatty acids help the brain direct nutrients to various body organs including the skin, to strengthen hair and nails, and to produce the required hormones and nerve impulses throughout the body. Sources – nuts, seeds, legumes, grains and herbs, or animal sources, fish, chicken, meats, eggs, yogurt, and cheese.

Micronutrients

Vitamins - a group of micronutrients that cannot be made by the body and must be obtained from our food, except for vitamin D which can be manufactured by the body when we are exposed to sunlight.

Vitamins that are water soluble cannot be stored by the body and need to be consumed every day. These include many B group vitamins and vitamin C. The fat-soluble vitamins A, D, E and K can be temporarily stored in fats we consume until required.

Vitamins act as coenzymes and assist enzymes in the formation of hormones, immunity and are used in cell production throughout the body. Vitamin deficiency is something you want to avoid, as it can result in loss of vital force within the body. A wholesome variety of fresh foods will provide the necessary vitamins for good health.

Vitamin A - good vision, reproduction, and the formation and maintenance of skin, mucous membranes, bones, and teeth. Sources - dark green leafy vegetables (collards, kale, spinach), yellow and orange fruits, vegetables, and animal products.

Vitamin B - mixture of eight essential vitamins necessary to enhance immune and nervous system function and promote cell growth and division. Sources - nuts, seeds, mushrooms, legumes, brewer's yeast, lean meats, eggs, leafy green vegetables, whole grains, and berries.

Vitamin C - powerful antioxidant, regulates blood pressure, blood pH, assists iron absorption, assists immune response and memory. Sources – citrus, tomatoes, capsicum, and peppers

Vitamin D - maintain bone, muscle, and cell health, aids calcium and phosphorus absorption. Source – sunshine, supplements, see Pat 1 environmental influences, section on sunshine.

Vitamin E - antioxidant, supports cell health and longevity. Sources – nuts, seeds, fruits, and vegetables.

Vitamin K - assists blood clotting, kidney, and bone health. Sources – eat your greens!

Minerals

Minerals – essential for human health, they are classified into two groups, main minerals, and trace minerals.

The main minerals are used in large quantities throughout the body. These are calcium, chloride, magnesium, phosphorus, potassium, sodium, and sulphur. The trace minerals are required in trace amounts, and include chromium, copper, fluoride, iodine, iron, lithium, manganese, molybdenum, selenium, and zinc. Minerals are essential to the function of enzymes, bones, blood, and overall cell health. With a balanced wholesome food intake, as suggested, you will meet your macro and micronutrient needs.

Calcium - is to build and help maintain strong bones and teeth, assists to regulate blood pressure, muscle contraction, nerve impulses and the blood. Sources – dairy products, seeds, nuts, fish, most leafy green vegetables.

Chloride - important electrolyte for the blood, electrical impulses from the brain, regulates blood volume pH and pressure, and cell fluid balance. Sources – sea salt, sea vegetables, olives, and salad.

Chromium - helps cells draw energy from the blood, maintains normal blood sugar levels, assists fats, protein, and carbohydrate metabolism. Sources – broccoli, grapes vegetables and poultry.

Copper - mopping up free radicals, assists with metabolism, red cell production and regulating neurotransmitters, immune system, skin, and bone health. Sources – seafood, meats, oats, dark chocolate, nuts, and seeds.

Iodine - supports thyroid function and hormone production to control metabolism, and cognitive function. Sources – sea vegetables, sea food, dairy products, eggs, legumes, and sea salt.

Iron - activates enzymes for amino acids, collagen, neurotransmitters, and hormones, assists to make haemoglobin (oxygen-transport chemical in red blood cells) and myoglobin (protein in muscle cells). Sources – seeds, nuts, legumes, grains, and red meat.

Lithium - mood regulation and mental health. Sources – nuts, seeds, grains vegetables, meats, and seafood.

Magnesium - assists to build bones and teeth, assists to regulate blood pressure, muscle contraction, enzymes, nerve impulses, blood sugar and clotting. Sources – seeds, grains, nuts, and green vegetables.

Manganese - helps bone formation, amino acids, cholesterol, and carbohydrate metabolism. Sources – seeds nuts, seafood, legumes, and vegetables.

Molybdenum - sulphite regulation by breaking down toxins through enzyme activation. Sources – legumes, nuts, grains, and leafy green vegetables.

Phosphorus - assists to build bones and teeth, assists fats, protein, and carbohydrate metabolism. Sources – legumes, nuts, meat, and dairy products.

Potassium - muscle contraction, fluid balance within the body. Sources – bananas, raisins, tomatoes, legumes, and root vegetables.

Selenium - brain function and supports immune system. Sources – brazil nuts, brown rice, and eggs.

Sodium - muscle contraction, nerve impulses, fluid balance within the body. Sources – sea salt, and most processed products.

Sulphur - food metabolism, cell genetic expression, and repair DNA. Sources – legumes, grains, seafood, meat, dairy, eggs, and green vegetables.

Zinc - helps blood clot, helps synthesise proteins and DNA for cell division, blood clotting, boost immunity, and wound healing. Sources – seeds, nuts, grains, seafood (oysters), meat, eggs.

Herbs & Spices

When considering taking herbal remedies, it is wise to consult a trained naturopath or herbalist. The use of herbs and spices in food preparation has been used for thousands of years and provides an excellent source of many micronutrients required for maintaining good health. If you are unsure how to use a particular herb or spice, do your research. This book glosses over some that are worth exploring further for 2020 and beyond.

Ashwagandha - (Indian Ginseng) stimulates white blood cell production and assists the immune system.

Cinnamon - contains cinnamaldehyde, an anti-bacterial and anti-viral, assisting the immune system.

Echinacea - helps encourage healthy cell growth, promotes a strong upper respiratory system, and provides numerous antioxidants to stimulate the immune system.

Elderberry - note the stems, leaves and roots are toxic. The flowers and berries contain anthocyanidins which also support the immune system and are anti-inflammatory.

Garlic - a pungent bulb containing allicin, with potent anti-bacterial, anti-viral and anti-fungal properties.

Ginger - a rhizome containing sesquiterpenes, stimulates immune response to infections and virus.

Ginseng - specifically Panax ginseng, is high in antioxidants, boosts the immune system and respiratory system.

Oregano - leaves and flowers are edible, with a pungent savory flavour with antibacterial, and antioxidant properties.

Turmeric - a rhizome, containing curcumin, which is an anti-inflammatory, and stimulates immune response to infections.

Part 3 – Psychological
Influences of the Mind

Part 3 – Psychological Influences of the Mind

Thoughts are very powerful things. Philosophers, scientists, and theologians throughout history have been pondering, debating, and discovering the true power and potential of our thoughts. They are all in complete agreement on one thing - we become what we think about.

This knowledge can be confronting the first time we hear it, especially if life isn't going the way we want it to; but once we understand the workings of our mind, it creates a marvellous awakening to our true nature, possibilities, and potential.

We live in a time of conflicting ideas that challenge who we are and what we believe. The brain is the instrument of the mind. Our body is directed by the brain, and we use our body to get things done in the physical world. We use our body to interact with others and the people we love in the physical world. Our body is a tool of the mind and when we are thinking in the present, the body is directed by the conscious mind to act in accordance with the values and beliefs held in the subconscious mind. When our conscious mind wanders or thinks of past events or even future events, our subconscious mind directs the body. One of the greatest challenges we face is to live in the present.

When we look past culture, learnt values, beliefs, physical or mental abilities, people are essentially the same. It is therefore our culture, values, beliefs, and abilities that make each of us unique. With the caveat of the preceding sentence, I am yet to meet a person that does not want happiness, health, love, and sufficient resources to carry out the essential needs and wants of life. We all have a mind with incalculable capacity and a body that reacts or responds to its environments and Ruling Mental State (RMS). Our current persona is a product of our culture, habitual beliefs, and values, and until we personally decide what we want, we remain like a cork in the ocean having the programmed paradigms from our youth, and our outside world inundate us with information, controlling how we think, act and live.

We all believe and perceive some things differently, so we need to try to understand where each of us is coming from, then we can be accepting of other beliefs and values without judgement. The concepts presented here are to create additional awareness, and with that awareness we can use our personal power to choose how we think, act and live.

Our minds need a purpose, positive loving relationships, and a sound belief system to function optimally. Cultivating these three psychological prerequisites will be explored in this section. We all require these three prerequisites so that our brain can direct the body to satisfy the natural environmental health influences and obtain and satisfy the biological needs of the physical body for the benefit of the whole. They are prerequisites for health, as they are fundamental laws that govern the effective use of the mind.

Purpose

Have you ever set a goal, or created a list of things you want to do in your life? Have you felt that you have a purpose for living on this small planet? Have you discovered your purpose? It behoves us to ponder and think until we discover our purpose.

When we discover our purpose, it will get us out of bed each day with enthusiasm to work toward achieving it. If we fail to find purpose and we are not in complete control of our mind, we will to a large extent, be controlled by our external environment, and the thoughts and desires of others.

This can create a mental conflict, as most people have a general idea of the things they like and wish to do, but without purpose the controlling forces of others will relentlessly act on us, often without our consent. Purpose is a fundamental law; either we act of our own will and desire or we will be acted upon. If we do not fill our time with our purpose, all our extra time will be filed with the desires and the controlling forces of others.

Our minds need direction

Our mind needs direction, goals, and a reason to grow. We need to be passionate about something; when we find that something, we have our purpose. From our purpose we create a vision in our conscious mind of how we can go about fulfilling our purpose, then we put our conscious mind to work to create a plan to make it happen. This is where two important facilities of the conscious mind, imagination, and the will, are required. When we find our purpose, we will likely become emotionally involved in the purpose. Research suggests becoming emotionally involved in our purpose is the most effective way to implant the purpose into the subconscious mind.

If you do not feel you can become emotionally involved in your purpose yet, that is OK. There are other ways of handing your purpose over to your subconscious mind. Write down your purpose, then create an affirmation around your purpose - a written note you can read to yourself when you wake up in the morning and read again before you go to bed at night. You may like to develop a vision board that you can view, as you do for your written affirmation.

When we have a plan and it is implanted in our subconscious mind to the extent that we think about it daily, our habits will begin to align with the plan, and this motivates and moves us into action. When we act, whether it be on our desires, or the desires of others, we get a result. The results or consequences follow laws. If the result is what we want, the result will give us confidence in our plan and capacity, and in time bring us to our goal. If the result is not what we want, it is because the action taken was not correct or was being partially or completely controlled by others or the immediate environment.

The preceding statements can be hard to swallow if this is the first time you have heard this. There is a law of cause and effect. In life we aim to control the causes we set in motion, so that we get the desired effects, conditions, circumstances, or results.

To find our passion, we might have to work at it for a while. We need to think about what we love to do and what comes easily to us. The things we find easiest to do, we already have programs for in our subconscious mind. If these things that we do by habit are good and contribute to our wellbeing and the wellbeing of those around us, we might be closer to finding our purpose than we think.

The challenge comes when we find things we do already, that come easily by habit, violate natural laws, causing us and those around us pain and suffering. If this is you, take heart; it is how most people operate until they learn the laws well enough to develop new habits.

New habits that are not in harmony with our paradigms often cause a conflict between our conscious mind that wants to adopt the new habit and our subconscious mind that is fixed with the old habits and does not want to change. This is covered in how to use the faculties of conscious mind later on.

Most of us have habits that run from our subconscious mind that are not even ours, as they were put directly into our subconscious mind in our first six years of life, before we developed the faculties and filters of the conscious mind.

The increased awareness that come with understanding these laws and how our mind works will help develop the power of thought necessary for us to discover our true purpose.

Ask yourself, what would you do if you had more than enough money so that you did not need to work for a living? What would you do if you knew you could not fail? These questions really get us thinking, because we all need to work at some time, and we all fail at some time. The key is to never give up, even when we eventually discover our purpose.

Nature's purpose is continuous growth, increase, and expansion. When something in our natural environment stops growing, it decays, and its energy is transferred to growth somewhere else. This is also true of our mind and body. Without passion we lack a reason to grow and expand; without growth and expansion the mind directs the brain to decay, a systematic apoptosis, and break down the body.

Positive Loving Relationships

The greatest of all emotions is love. Without love, the mind sees no reason to grow and expand. In the Greek language there are three kinds of love, and positive loving relationships can be found in all three:

- **Eros** - Romantic love for a spouse or partner, sexual passion and desire, originating after the Greek god of fertility.
- **Philia** - Deep friendship love, a loyal love, a comradely love, sacrifice and sharing emotions, the love a parent has for a child, partner, sibling, relative, parent, or close friend.
- **Agape** - Selfless love, this love of humanity, friends, partner, family, or strangers, from a biblical translation to Latin we have caritas, which is charity, or the pure love of Christ.

There is also a need for self-love; not a self-obsessed, self-centred love, but a healthier love for self that enhances our capacity to love others.

The ancient Greeks tried to nurture all the loves with balance. This is what is meant by positive loving relationships and why it makes the list of pre-requisites for health. Positive loving relationships help us to feel good about ourselves and others and improves our outlook of the world.

We are all connected

We are all connected to one another through vibratory forces that are not widely understood. This vibratory force is also known as frequency, or cycles of a wave of energy that pass a point in one second. The higher the frequency the greater the energy. It is important to realise that nothing rests, everything is oscillating at a frequency all the time. When we connect with someone, we have a thought that is on the same frequency, we resonate, just like two tuning forks across a room.

This connected vibration is most obvious when we are laughing. Laughter is contagious. Try an experiment, where you think about an event you can recall that was really funny, that nobody around you at the time knows anything about. As you focus your mind on the funny event, you move onto that frequency and start laughing. As you get going with a good belly laugh, people in close proximity to you will begin to laugh too, and the more you laugh the more others close by will start laughing, without even knowing what you are laughing about. If you do this for a while, some may start laughing hysterically, all because you have created a laughter vibration that they have felt internally that is causing them to laugh.

Humour and laughter that come at the expense of others, may provide short term enjoyment, for a few. This will rarely catch on as in the experiment above because the vibration created may be mixed and varied. When we have a hearty laugh with people, that does not hurt others, the body moves into a synchronised positive vibration with the whole group. This laughter vibration from a collective group of people provides increased health benefits, proportional to the size of the group.

The connected vibration is often experienced in close relationships when we finish our partner's sentence for them. Other times we may be thinking about a friend who is interstate or overseas; then our phone rings and it is them on the other end of the line. This is not coincidence, this happens by law. We put a vibration out there, that penetrates time and space; they feel the frequency and decide to make the call.

Through relationships one feels a sense of belonging. Relationships are somewhere we can share our values and similarities without judgement or criticism, allowing one to feel unconditionally loved. We all need to belong somewhere, whether a sporting, community, cultural, gardening, musical, religious, service, or workplace group.

When we feel we do not belong, we may want to explore our environment and our surroundings to find the source of that feeling. Recognising the source of that feeling creates personal awareness and this is the first step to discovering where we fit, and this empowers us to find others with similar ideas and values.

The feeling of belonging increases self-love, self-worth and forms positive loving relationships. These positive loving relationships increase energy output and cause positive hormones to be released into the body, bringing vibrant mental clarity and a deep richness to life that can be found in no other way.

Belief system

A belief system is first formed from our parents, early carers and by our early influences. These initial beliefs are our paradigms. A paradigm is nothing more than a multitude of learned habits that are carried out by our subconscious mind without our knowledge, control, or consent for the rest of our lives. Research suggests these early paradigms may provide the controlling forces that underpin all our major decisions.

Research on the workings of the subconscious mind also suggest these paradigms can be shaped and modified by our life experiences, when coupled with an intense emotional experience. However, in the absence of an intense emotional experience or persistent repetition, we are unlikely to vary from these controlling paradigms throughout of our lives.

Some of us have been programmed with very strong beliefs in a higher force, greater than oneself - God, Universal Intelligence, The Great Spirit, the Sixth Sense, or Natural Laws of the Universe. Unfortunately, many of us do not know what to believe. With confusion and contradictions all around, we may reach adulthood without developing a belief system. Sometimes long held beliefs are shattered as described above by an intense emotional experience.

I grew up with some token Christian values from my parents; my father who was Greek Orthodox, and my mother was Presbyterian. As I grew up, I did not accept these beliefs, largely due to contradictions I observed between beliefs and behaviour. It is not my place to judge; however, I observed enough as I was growing up to know religion was not for me, although I did feel a weak connection to a higher power or God.

One of my firm beliefs as I grew older, is that there is a God with an organised purpose who governs and set the laws that are explored in this book. I am often asked, 'how could you as a scientist possibly ever believe in God?' Well, it is my belief in God that caused me to want to study science and to understand how our environments influence our health and wellbeing. I also believe that any self-help book such as this, that lacks a spiritual component, is incomplete.

I am grateful for my beliefs and when I consider one of the common theories regarding the origin of life on earth, I rationalise 'could an explosion in a printing press produce this book?' No, it comes from arranging and organising information. Everything around us in nature follows established and exacting laws that were set by someone. I am not trying to turn this into a religious dissertation; however, I want to make the point about belief. We all need to believe in something; it could be a belief in ourselves, a loved one, God, Jesus Christ, or a belief in our abilities. Whatever we choose to call this belief, make no mistake the energy created from belief is a force that is penetrating and impacting every cell in your body.

The foundation of belief is faith.

Faith is not to have a perfect knowledge of things; therefore, if we have faith, we hope for things which we cannot see, which we believe are true. For example, I have not seen God or Jesus Christ, however my belief makes them true to me. I am not going to go any deeper than this into my faith; suffice to say, many books have been written on faith and belief including the Bible and other teachings of Jesus Christ, if one wishes to explore this belief.

When we choose to examine our beliefs, regarding why we believe what we believe, we may be able to highlight beliefs that do not make any logical sense, or worse, cause us to compromise or violate the laws that govern our health and wellbeing. The best example of this that comes to mind is smoking cigarettes. Unfortunately, some time ago, a clever and sinister group of people discovered tobacco, which contained a highly addictive substance called nicotine. They plotted and schemed ways they could convince the believing public, that smoking cigarettes was actually good for them. It worked, and now there are more than fifteen billion cigarettes smoked each day around the world. We do not really need a medical study or scientific evidence to tell us that smoking cigarettes and inhaling a cocktail of poisonous gases, is not doing us any favours. It is preventing our bodies from satisfying the law that states our bodies require clean air to function correctly.

In truth, there are literally thousands of examples of beliefs that destroy the health of our bodies or take away our free agency and our ability to live the lives we truly want. This was another huge motivator for me writing this book. Clever marketers who understand this law perfectly, use it to their advantage with absolute exactness, to lay waste the lives of millions who do not fully comprehend the power of this law of belief.

This is where the will comes in. If you think that these nine laws described in this book are true, and by the way they are true, you are now empowered to change some incorrect beliefs you may have been carrying all your life. The persistent use of the will; the will being one of the faculties of the conscious mind. Our will, when applied repeatedly and with persistence, ensures the old beliefs held that may have been found to be incorrect, can actually be changed and overwritten with new beliefs and impressions.

With persistence, the new impressions planted in the subconscious mind become stronger than the old habits. The old habits do not disappear; however, they do become weaker. The new habits take the place of the old habits as a new routine played by the subconscious mind. When these new habits are acted on through correct application of the new beliefs, a cause is set in motion, and the effect comes by law.

When the new habits are formed and applied daily, the body can heal itself and restore balance. This may take time, as cells in the body are replaced at different rates; however, with consistent application of the nine laws of health over time, the resulting feeling of wellbeing will become increasingly rapid. This is not magic; it is happening by the law of cause and effect. The body healing itself and coming into balance is what gives the vibrant health, fitness, and abundant energy you can often observe in many young and also some very old people.

Learned habitual influences.

Many of us carry habits that influence our values, beliefs, behaviour, and health to such an extent, that this information is simply too much to comprehend and apply. We may learn these new truths and when we try to apply them, the old programs playing in our subconscious mind cause us to reject this information, despite the fact we want to change and regain our health and wellbeing.

We may need to unlearn and relearn new habits, and it is through an understanding and awareness of these laws on a superficial level in our conscious mind that we can develop the tools to unlearn and relearn. We can use the faculties of the conscious mind to reason, examine, evaluate, and rationalise the new information. Most of the information is not really new, it has just been mixed with so much confusion and contradiction that is has become difficult to see clearly.

This confusing information has been mixed in our past with old habits that are likely not even of our choosing. It is the awareness and the plain speaking within this book that can make all the difference. I encourage you to get to know your mind, and how your mind influences your brain to create vibrations and chemicals that are of your choosing, that can be released into your body that will lead to wellbeing. The technical section that follows is specifically included to help you do that.

Technical Information – Subconscious and Conscious Mind

What is the brain made of?

There are approximately 160,000 km of blood vessels, 100 billion neurons, that can perform ten quadrillion (million billion) operations per second.

In the brain one million cells die and are replaced every second, with this kind of activity some neurologists believe the potential neural connection is limitless.

The adult brain weighs between 1.2 to 1.5 kg and is about 1.5% of body weight.

The brain uses the following proportion of the resources of the body to function normally.

- 20% air we breathe,
- 25% of the blood flow,
- 30% of water intake,
- 40% of nutrient from blood stream,

The brain has both grey and white matter. The grey matter is made up of neurons that gather and transmit signals, while the white matter is made of dendrites and axons that the neurons use to transmit signals.

The brain is composed of approximately:

- 78% water,
- 10% lipids (fat),
- 8% protein,
- 1% carbohydrate,
- 2% soluble organics,
- 1% inorganic salts.

Your brain is really the central processing unit (CPU), or electronic switching station and chemist, for the vibrations that it picks up via your senses of sight, sound, smell, taste, touch and intuition or gut feeling. The brain then sends the electrical impulses and chemical compounds to where they are required to perform the functions of the body.

Look after your brain and it will manage your body systems well; this will go a long way towards maintaining perfect lifelong health. If you have ever experienced brain fog, headache, or loss of mental clarity, look at your water consumption (refer section on water).

Workings of the Mind

Parameter	Conscious Brain	Subconscious Brain
Mass	17%	83%
Impulse Speed	200 - 250 km/h	over 160,000 km/h
Bits of information processed per second	2000	400,000,000 +
Control of perception and behaviour	2 - 4%	96 - 98%
Function	Volitional	Servile
Time	Past, Present and Future	Present
Memory	up to 20 seconds	Forever
Inputs	Subconscious Mind, 5 Senses	Conscious Mind, 6th Sense
Outputs	Physical Communication	Vibrations, Impulses, Paradigms

The mind directs the brain to produce electrical impulses and manufacture chemical compounds. These chemical compounds and electrical impulses are sent to every organ and cell in the body so that the body's autonomic systems will function without conscious intervention. Further, these chemical compounds and electrical impulses are sent by the brain to direct movement functions that will be in direct accordance with the desires of the RMS of the mind, and the body will correspondingly experience the emotions of the RMS. This is how our thinking influences where we choose to spend our time, the environment we live in, and our social networks, and consequently this then determines to a large extent our mental health.

The Subconscious Mind

The subconscious mind only lives in the present, and it never sleeps, remembers absolutely everything, has absolutely no sense of humour, cannot differentiate between what is imagined and what is real.

The subconscious mind processes all new information and based on our conscious choices and decisions files this information in accordance with beliefs, values, and habits.

One of the problems experienced by the vast majority of people is negativity about their capacity. Let me explain; by the age of about sixteen years when many of us finish school we have been told "no you can't" an estimated 140,000 times or 24 times each day since we were born. Depending on your school and parents, you may have also been told "no, you are not good enough" a few thousand times as well, over the same period of time.

Consider by the same age where you have been told "yes you can" only an estimated 5,000 times - less than once a day since birth. People tend to grow up with an inferiority complex and truly believe they cannot do something or are not good enough to even set and achieve goals.

When we consider 96 to 98% of our behaviour is habitual and automatic, it becomes easier to see why conditioning the subconscious mind is so important to living an abundant life of joy, happiness, loving relationships, health, and prosperity. It is also interesting to note that the same percentage of people, 96 to 98%, do not have well defined written down goals, that they act on as a matter of habit.

Harvard University researchers carried out a study of human potential over a 20-year period. The researchers found that those that had clearly defined written goals that were acted upon, accounted for 3% of those that took part in the study. After 20 years they found this 3% were healthier and generally happier than the rest of the participants. Further, the combined net worth of that 3% was greater than the combined entire net worth of the other 97% of those involved in the study.

The point I'm making here is the subconscious mind is the driving force that needs to be directed. If you will give it a task, and plant it deep enough to form a habit, watch it magically bring you everything you want in life including great health.

Our subconscious mind is constantly working without our knowledge or control. You may be driving your car - are you really driving, or is your subconscious mind driving?

Once you have learnt to drive, this is happening on auto pilot, unless someone cuts you off or there is an event that gets your attention; then in a split second your conscious mind takes control, and you act based on the information picked up by your senses. Then as soon as the event passes, you go back to autopilot.

A good example of this is when you are driving; your passenger says something like 'remember last week when we were at the beach'? You do not suddenly stop driving so you can go back in time to last week when you were at the beach; your conscious mind goes back, and your subconscious drives the car. This is the same when you think of a future event, your conscious mind travels to the future event and your subconscious mind drives the car.

> **"Time travel is reserved for the conscious mind. The subconscious mind lives in the present"**

You get a glimpse of the enormity and capacity of your mind when you hear a quote from Dr. Emanuel Donchin, director of the Laboratory for Cognitive Psychophysiology at the University of Illinois.

> **" An enormous portion of cognitive activity is non-conscious, figuratively speaking, it could be 99 percent; we probably will never know precisely how much is outside awareness."**

The subconscious mind contains paradigms learnt from before we were born. When we were in the womb, we felt our parents and surroundings, the vibrations, and emotions of those around us. Then when we were born this continued; we had not yet developed the faculties of the conscious mind or how to use the five senses to filter.

We were programmed genetically, receiving the genetic imprint from our parents, a logical reason why we often look like our parents. Then we were subject to every feeling, conversation, input from radio, TV, news, games, the internet, and people we may not have even known.

They filled our subconscious mind with information. The information that came in often enough, created a pattern or program that then became a habitual thought. By the time we had developed the filtering faculties of our conscious mind to the extent where we could effectively filter, accept, or reject information, we had been programmed - programmed with a multitude of habits, beliefs and values that form our self-image. This all happened by the time we reached five or six years old. Most of these paradigms were being learnt and became habitual routines well before our conscious faculties fully developed. Some of these paradigms are not of our choosing, with many passed down from our parents and early influences.

Through an increased awareness and an understanding of our paradigms, we can create an awareness that will allow us to do almost anything. A reliable estimate of the currently utilised portions of the human mind is five to ten percent of its capacity. That said, if we could use fifty percent of our minds we could learn and speak, read, and write forty languages, memorise the entire Encyclopedia Britannica cover to cover and complete many doctorates with distinction. For all intents and purposes, the potential of the human mind is limitless, only limited by our imagination and paradigms.

The subconscious mind can process 400,000,000 bits of information per second both night and day; however only information that is in harmony with our paradigms is delivered to the conscious mind to create our impression of the world. This is why some of us are experts in deletion and others seem to notice everything. It is funny listening to a close friend, who often reminds me of things that I missed. Our subconscious mind determines which of the 2000 bits of information coming in each second are noticed, accepted, or rejected and deleted. For example, when you enter a venue what do you notice? The happy couple laughing and talking over a meal, the person sitting on their own staring at the painting on the wall, or the couple arguing with the waiter. The subconscious mind cannot differentiate between the real and imaginary world, it perceives all and on-delivers to the conscious mind what is in harmony with its learned paradigms.

What does this have to do with our environment, our social and mental health? The first part of the process is to recognise that our thoughts are energy in motion, and these thoughts create vibrations that we interpret as feelings. Intense feelings impress on the subconscious mind and form new habits, and when the emotion is strong enough and brought to the conscious mind repeatedly, it forms a new paradigm in the subconscious mind. Paradigms are formed and changed in three other ways - hypnosis, repetition, and auto suggestion. Neurolinguistic Programming (NLP) has been around for a few decades and incorporates all of the above to some extent. There is research being done to accelerate subconscious paradigm shifts, suggesting reprogramming can be done in a matter of minutes.

99

"To be able to shape your future you have to be willing to change your paradigm." **Joel Barker**

We create our environment.

We think thoughts, and these thoughts cause us to act in a certain way. Once we act, we set a cause in motion; then through the natural laws that govern our world, all causes have an effect; that effect is, put simply, a consequence. We only need to look at the state of our rivers, air quality in our cities and buildings, the state of our farmlands and ecosystems to see the consequences of our actions.

Likewise, we can see other beautiful consequences with the advances in medicine, technology, and our built environments. We have created, to a large extent, the environments we choose to live in through our own thoughts and actions.

The same is true for our social environments; what we think and believe determines who we associate with, what we think and value, determines what we say, and the cycle continues with a consequence. Our environments that we create, and our social interactions that we choose, to a large extent determine our state of mental health and therefore wellbeing.

How do we control the paradigms that govern why we think, say, and do the things we do, react the way we do, buy the things we buy and ultimately believe what we believe? When we were young, we didn't know what we didn't know, so we often did whatever was in harmony with our dominant paradigms.

> **"**
> *"When you look at a person – you can often see, are they healthy, happy, loved, wealthy – results tell the truth."* **Roy Stanford**

Faculties of the conscious mind

The conscious mind is our creative mind receiving inputs from our five senses; we see, hear, smell, taste and touch our environment. We have thoughts and ideas coming in through our senses, and our subconscious mind causes us to filter these thoughts and impulses, based on our perception of our beliefs and values, our sixth sense (gut feeling) and our emotions. We are actually deleting most of the amazing 2000 bits of information the conscious mind can process each second.

We all need to create awareness of some of the controlling forces in our lives so that we can look after our mind. We use our conscious mind to think and reason why our paradigms cause us to think and believe as we do. A paradigm is nothing more than a multitude of learned habits that we use to filter the world around us. These paradigms also make us do and think the way we do; therefore, we can change any or all of them with conscious effort, as described above in the section on the subconscious mind.

The conscious mind is where our will power comes from. It can travel to the past and future; when it comes back to the present, it can originate ideas, plan and create new things, and change paradigms. Everything you see around you, besides nature and space, has been created first in the conscious mind, with definite plans to bring the thought to a tangible reality.

The conscious mind can think, reason, and therefore accept or reject the ideas of others; however, in the absence of active response thought, our acceptance or rejection of ideas will be based on our paradigms. For example, you might be reading this, and your impulsive reaction may be to either accept it as fact or reject it as a bunch of nonsense.

In the presence of active response thought, reasoning, and an understanding of the law, you may respond by developing your opinion about the subject matter and choose to plant your conclusion in your subconscious mind.

Our conscious mind is easily distracted through our senses. We can go into the past in an instant, or into a future planned event, but this is ok because our subconscious mind is doing the rest, as explained before with driving the car, or walking, cycling, eating, and running; the subconscious is running thousands of processes of the body.

Our environment is so important to our psychological wellbeing. When your environment is clean, uncluttered, supportive, loving, and orderly the conscious mind can do what it does best - create and originate ideas, learn new things, and experience the wonders all around.

A fatalistic view of life is often the result of our programming and environment. We may have been told we have bad genes, we are not smart enough, we may have been exposed to violence, abuse, drugs, or chemicals and believe our lot in life is fixed and there is nothing we can do about it. This is not true; there is evidence that even our genes are subject to our environment. Scientific discoveries during the last century have revealed how large a role our mind and environment play in determining our wellbeing.

I briefly introduced the term epigenetics, in the whole food section back in Part 2. Epigenetics is the study of heritable changes in gene expression (active versus inactive genes) that do not involve changes to the underlying DNA sequence — a change in phenotype without a change in genotype — which in turn affects how cells read the genes.

A Japanese scientist Kazuhiro Sakurada stated "Techniques for controlling epigenetic modification by environmental factors may also play a critical role in the development of epigenetically stable sources of pluripotent stem cells. Pluripotent bone marrow stem cell capable of giving rise to many different cell types."

Kazuhiro's theory was proven true by Dr. Bruce Lipton, a stem cell biologist at Stamford University, and a lecturer at Wisconsin School of Medicine. He conducted an experiment with stem cells, where he extracted a stem cell from a human and cultured it in a growth medium in a petri dish. A cell will divide in ten hours and in a little over a week there will be 50,000 plus cells, Lipton divided them into three petri dishes and changed the culture, then grew muscle cells in one, fat cells in another and bone cells in the third dish.

Dr Lipton concluded that cellular perceptions of the environment are the primary factor in our biological processes; our cells are responding to their environment, then regulate cell transcription based on the cellular environment. The cellular environment in the body that regulates gene expression is the blood. When you think about it, we as humans are really a skin covered petri dish, as Lipton puts it. As discussed previously, the mind directs the brain which is the chemist that creates the chemicals and the vibratory frequency of the body. From this you can see how important it is to control your thoughts and the paradigms that run in the subconscious mind.

The gene is the blueprint of life; the mind, and the environment it creates through the brain, control the development of the 100,000 protein chains made in the body, and therefore cells' gene expression. The mind can direct the brain to produce hormones based on our mood expression from our habitual thoughts or RMS of mind. For example, the happy hormones dopamine, oxytocin, serotonin, and endorphins.

Alternatively, our mind can direct the brain to produce stress hormones - Adrenaline, Cortisol, Norepinephrine. These stress chemicals shut off the immune system to conserve energy for flight or fight. This is our mind effectively shutting down the immune system, our body's defences, allowing the body to become susceptible to disease.

The compounds that are manufactured by our brain affect every cell and system in the body. A hormone imbalance can be debilitating. Some signs that may indicate you could be making stress chemicals and your hormones are out of balance, are bloating, fatigue, irritability, hair loss, palpitations, mood swings, problems with blood sugar, trouble concentrating. If you experience any of these symptoms, seek advice from your medical doctor to treat the acute symptoms and then learn how to manage your mind.

Problems often start when the conscious mind learns something new, tries to do it and finds it difficult or impossible. This is because it is not the conscious mind doing the new thing; this is the job of the subconscious mind. Therefore, if the paradigm in the subconscious mind is not in harmony with the values and beliefs of the new thing, you will not do it. Why? Because there is a conflict, as stated earlier, remembering the subconscious is operating at hundreds of times the capacity of the conscious mind. The subconscious mind will win every time. The subconscious mind plays the paradigm, which is nothing more than a series of habits that are formed in our mind that almost exclusively control our habitual behaviours. Paradigms also have the capacity to control our perception.

Our thoughts create feelings that can be good or bad and produce the good or bad result. Any thoughts you repeatedly hold, whether a new thought or an existing program or habitual thought, running from your subconscious mind will eventually create your reality. Thoughts are things and when mixed with the emotions created by the subconscious mind, lead our bodies into action; the actions bring a consequence, and the consequence, whether good or bad, is often in harmony with our deepest beliefs.

If our results are in harmony with our paradigm this will give us confidence; this increases our belief and faith in our ability, which creates more good feelings, and the cycle continues.

Sometimes we learn something new and we like what we hear, despite it being new information; the new information is in conflict with our paradigm. As long as we do not act on the new information and it stays in our conscious mind, nothing happens, and our subconscious mind continues to play its programs unchallenged.

If you really like the new information and decide to act on it - reading this book for example - the subconscious becomes involved and the conflict starts; and we experience emotions of worry, fear, and anxiety, because of the conflicting paradigm, so we tend to do nothing and move back or retreat to the comfort of the old paradigm. This processing happens at the speed of thought, which is akin to the speed of light, maybe even faster; we do not really know how fast our thoughts travel. This is why some people have read every self-help book out there and nothing changes.

This can be the prime cause of mental conflict, anxiety, frustration, and fear that often lead to depression and other mental health issues; this can also lead to drug abuse and dependency, as a means of escape from the conflict between the two minds. Have you ever heard anyone say, "they are in two minds about something?"

We learn, but we often do not do what we now want to do, or know we should do with the new knowledge, because the paradigms that run in our subconscious mind are controlling our actions. You could say this can lead to superior knowledge but inferior results. Almost all our behaviours are habitual; we need to be able to learn, unlearn, and then relearn new habits that will give us what we want. Once you change the old paradigm, the change can be permanent.

If you want to change paradigms that are not serving you, first you need to recognise what you are feeling, and then you will know what chemical and hormones your brain is making and distributing into your blood stream, affecting all the new cells that are being made every second of every day.

Some sure ways to get your brain making the good chemicals are laughing, having a long hug, some intimacy, spending time with people you love, meditating to calm down, completing a goal, setting some new goals, treating your senses, good smells, tasty and healthy food, getting some sunshine, fresh air, exercise and drinking more water, getting plenty of rest, satisfying the nine laws of health each day.

School gave us knowledge and so did our tertiary studies, but nobody routinely teaches us how to alter our old paradigms, which ultimately control our lives.

"

"in the absence of clearly defined goals we become strangely loyal to performing daily trivia, until we ultimately become enslaved by it" **Robert Heinlein**

"do just once what others say you can't do, and you will never pay attention to their limitations again." Captain James Cook

To bring all the nine laws together, we learn to respect ourselves, honour the great gift of life, use our body wisely which allows us to innovate, create and fulfil the measure of our creation. When we are responsible for our actions, we are happier, healthier, and more grateful.

My goal here is to help others set worthy goals and enjoy the journey to progressively realise those goals. Our belief, love and passion for life will spark our imagination, taking us to worlds yet to be created; however, without these physiological attributes, we go nowhere.

For more information on how our environment and thoughts are creating our wellbeing, or how you can reprogram old paradigms to live the life you desire, visit wellbeingmanagement.com.au. You can also download the wellness app here.

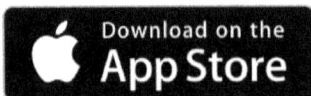

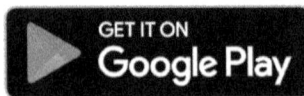

Bibliography

Allan, J (1903) *As A Man Thinketh*. Republished 2019 St Martin's Press. ISBN: 9781250309334.

Arner, P., Kriegholm, E., Engfeldt, P., Bolinder, J. (1990). *Adrenergic regulation of lipolysis in situ at rest and during exercise. J. Clin. Invest. 85.*

Augustin, L., Franceschi, S., Jenkins, D, et al. (2002). *Glycaemic index in chronic disease: a review.* European Journal of Clinical Nutrition.

Bagchi, D., Nair, S., Sen, C.K. (2019). *Nutrition and Enhanced Sports Performance: Muscle Building, Endurance, and Strength*. London: Academic Press.

Ballor, D.L., McCarthy, J.P., Wilterdink, E.J. (1990). *Exercise intensity does not affect the composition of diet and exercise-induced body mass loss*. American Journal Clinical Nutrition. 51.

Barker, J.A., Erickson, S.W. (2005). *Five Regions of the Future; Preparing your Business for Tomorrow's Technology Revolution*. Portfolio. ISBN: 1591840899.

Batmanghelidj, F. (1997). Your Body's Many Cries for Water. 2nd ed. Global Health Solutions, Inc. Vienna. ISBN: 0962994251.

Bijlsma, N. (2010). *Healthy Home Healthy Family. Is where you live affecting your health*. Queensland. Joshua Books. ISBN: 9780980179812.

Brown, S. (1992). *Vegetarian Cookbook*. London: Dorling Kindersley. ISBN: 0 86318 265 8.

Budwig, J. (2000). *Cancer: The Problem and the Solution*. Nexus Gmbh; 1 edition. ISBN: 978-3981050219.

Campbell, N.A. (1996). Biology. ,4th ed. The Benjamin Cummings Publishing Company, Inc California. ISBN: 0805319573.

Chu, C., Simpson, R. (1994). *Ecological Public Health: From Vision to Practice*. Watson Ferguson & Company. Queensland. ISBN: 0868575526.

Clark, M., Reed, D.B., Crouse, S.F., Armstrong, R.B. (2003). *Pre- and post-season dietary intake, body composition, and performance indices of NCAA division I female soccer players.* Int J Sport Nutrition Exercise Metabolism. September.

Costill, D.F., Coyle, E.F., Dalsky, G., Evans, W., Fink, W., Hoopes, D. (1977). *Effects of elevated plasma FFA and insulin on muscle glycogen usage during exercise.* J. Appl. Physiol. 43.

Coyle, E.F., Coggan, A.R., Hemmert, M.K., Lowe, R.C., Walters T.J. (1985). *Substrate usage during prolonged exercise following a pre-exercise meal.* J. Appl. Physiol. 59.

Deurenberg, P., Westrate, J.A., Seidell, J.C. (1991). *Body mass index as a measure of body fatness: age and sex prediction formulas.* Brit J Nutrition.

Duke, J.A. (1997). *The Green Pharmacy.* Rodale Press Pennsylvania. ISBN: 0875963161.

Dwyer J. (2006) *Harrisons Principles of Internal Medicine;* Nutritional Requirements and Dietary Assessment. USA: The McGraw-Hill Companies.

Essen, B., Hagenfeldt, L., Kaijser, L. (1977). *Utilization of blood-borne and intramuscular substrates during continuous and intermittent exercise in man.* J. Physiol. 265.

Farwell, L. A., Donchin, E. *"Talking off the top of your head: Toward a mental prosthesis utilizing event-related brain potentials,"* Electroencephalography. Clinical Neurophysiology, Vol 70.

Farrer, K.T.H. (1983). *Fancy Eating that: A closer look at food additives and contaminants.* Victoria: The Dominion Press Hedges & Bell. ISBN:0 522842437

Frankl,, V.E. (1946). *Man's Search For Meaning.* Austria. ISBN: 0671023373.

Gray, D.F. (1970). *Immunology* 2nd ed. F. W. Cheshire Publishing Victoria. SBN: 701505079.

Hoffman, J. (2019). *Dietary Supplementation in Sport and Exercise: Evidence, Safety and Ergogenic Benefits*. Milton Park, Abingdon, Oxon: Routledge.

Holliwell, R. (1939) *Working with the Law*. Republished 2005 DeVorss & Company. ISBN: 0875168086.

Horne, R. (1980). *The Health Revolution*, 5th edn. Sydney: Harper Collins Publishers. ISBN: 0 7322 5766 2

Hurley, B.F., Nemeth, P.M., Martin, W.H., Hagberg, J.M., Dalsky, G.P., Holloszy J.O. (1986). *Muscle triglyceride utilization during exercise: effect of training*. J. Appl. Physiol. 60.

International Atomic Energy Agency, Vienna. (1992). *Agrochemical: Fate in Food and the Environment*. IAEA Austria. ISBN: 9200103820.

Iraki, J., Fitschen, P., Espinar, S., Helms, E. (2019). *Nutrition recommendations for bodybuilders in the off-season*: A narrative review. Sports (Basel). June.

Issekutz, B., Paul, B. (1968). *Intramuscular energy sources in exercising normal and pancreatectomized dogs*. Am. J. Physiol. 215(1).

Jenner, S.L., Buckley, G.L., Belski, R., Devlin, B.L., Forsyth, A.K. (2019). *Dietary Intakes of Professional and Semi-Professional Team Sport Athletes Do Not Meet Sport Nutrition Recommendations* — A Systematic Literature Review. Nutrients. May.

Jensen, M.D., Caruso, M., Heiling, V., Miles, J.M. (1989). *Insulin regulation of lypolysis in nondiabetic and IDDM subjects*. Diabetes 38.

Jeukendrup, A.E., Saris, W.H.M., Schrauwen, P., Brouns, F., Wagenmakers, A.J.M (1995). *Metabolic availability of medium-chaim triglycerides coingested with carbohydrate during prolonged exercise*. J. Appl. Physiol. 79.

Kanter, M. (2018) *High-quality carbohydrates and physical performance: Expert panel report*. Nutrition Today. January.

Kiens, B., Essen-Gustavsson, B., Christensen, N.J., Saltin, B. (1993). *Skeletal muscle substrate utilization during submaximal exercise in man*. J. Physiol. (London) 469.

Klein, S., Coyle, E.F., Wolfe, R.R. (1994). *Fat metabolism during low-intensity exercise in endurance-trained and untrained men.* Am. J. Physiol. 267 (Endocrinol. Metab. 30).

Klapper, M.D. (1994). *A Diet for All Reasons.* This video was recorded in the United States of America and can be obtained through: Natural Health Society (NSW).

Lipton, B.H. (2015). *Biology of belief, Unleashing the Power of the Consciousness, Matter & Miracles*, Hay House Inc USA

Machado-Vieira, R., Manji, H. K., Zarate, C. A., Jr (2009). *The role of lithium in the treatment of bipolar disorder: convergent evidence for neurotrophic effects as a unifying hypothesis.* Bipolar disorders, 11 Suppl 2(Suppl 2).

MacFarlane, M., & Williams, A. C. (2004). *Apoptosis and disease: a life or death decision.* EMBO reports, 5(7).

McCabe, E. (1998). *O₂xygen Therapies.* Energy Publications Morrisville. ISBN: 0962052701.

Mackie, B.G., Dudley, G.A., Kaciuba-Uscilko, H., Terjung, R.L. (1980). *Uptake of chylomicron triglycerides by contracting skeletal muscle in rats.* J. Appl. Physiol. 49.

McKeith, G. (2000) *Living Food for Health.* London: Judy Piatkus Publishers Ltd. ISBN: 0 7499 2074 2

Martin, W.H., Dalsky, G.P., Hurley, B.F., Matthews, D.E., Bier, D.M., Hagberg, J.O., Holloszy, J.O. (1993). *Effect of endurance training on plasma FFA turnover and oxidation during exercise.* Am. J. Physiol. 265 (Endocrinol. Metab. 28).

Montain, S.J., Hopper, M.K., Coggan, A.R., Coyle, E.F. (1991). *Exercise metabolism at different time intervals after a meal.* J. Appl. Physiol. 70(2).

Morgan, T.E., Short, F.A., Cobb, L.A. (1969). *Effect of long-term exercise on skeletal muscle lipid composition.* Am. J. Physiol. 216.

Morton, R.W., Murphy, K.T., McKellar, S.R., Schoenfeld, B.J., et al. (2018). *A systematic review, meta-analysis and meta-regression of the effect of protein supplementation on resistance training-induced gains in muscle mass and strength in healthy adults.* Br Journal Sports Medicine. March.

Mosher, S.L., Sparks, S.A., Williams, E.L., Bentley, D.J., Mc Naughton, L.R. (2016). *Ingestion of a nitric oxide enhancing supplement improves resistance exercise performance.* J Strength Cond Res. December.

Natural Health Society of Australia. (1994-2020). *Vegetarian and Natural Health Magazines.* Phone (02) 4721 5068

Oscai, L.B., Essig, D.A., Palmer, W.K. (1990). *Lipase regulation of muscle triglyceride hydrolysis.* J. Appl. Physiol. 69.

Phinney, S.D., Bistrian, W.J., Evans, E., et al. (1983). *The human metabolic response to chronic ketosis without caloric restriction: preservation of submaximal exercise capability with reduced carbohydrate oxidation.* Metabolism 32.

Reidy, P.T., Rasmussen, B.B. (2016) *Role of ingested amino acids and protein in the promotion of resistance exercise-induced muscle protein anabolism.* Journal Nutrition. February.

Romijn, J.A., Coyle, E.F., Sidossis, L.S., Gastaldelli, A., Horowitz, J.F., et al. (1993). *Regulation of endogenous fat and carbohydrate metabolism in relation to exercise intensity and duration.* Am. J. Physiol. 265 (Endocrinol. Metab. 28).

Sakurada, K. (2010). *Environmental epigenetic modifications and reprogramming-recalcitrant genes.* Stem cell research. 4. 157-64.

Savory, A., Butterfield, J. (1999). *Holistic Management, A new Framework for Decision Making.* 2nd ed. Island Press, Washington. ISBN: 155963488.

Simonsen, J.C., Sherman, W.M., Lamb, D.R., Dernbach, A.R., Doyle, J.A., Strauss, R. (1991). *Dietary carbohydrate, muscle glycogen, and power during rowing training.* J. Appl. Physiol. 70.

Symmonds, E.M., Symmonds, I.M. (2004). *Essential Obstetrics & Gynaecology.* Spain: Churchill Livingstone; National Women's Health Centre, Nutrition.

Terjung, R. (1995). *Muscle adaptations to aerobic training.* Sports Sci. Exchange 8.

Terjung, R.L., Mackie, B.G., Dudley, G.A., Kaciuba-Uscilko, H. (1983). *Influence of exercise on chylomicron triacylglycerol metabolism: plasma turnover and muscle uptake.* Med. Sci. Sports Exercise.

Thomas, D.T., Erdman, K.A., Burke, L.M. (2016) *Position of the Academy of Nutrition and Dietetics,* Dietitians of Canada, and the American College of Sports Medicine: Nutrition and athletic performance. J Academy Nutrition Dietetics. March.

Thompson, C.D., Chisolm, A., Mclachlan, S.K., Campbell, J.M. (2008). *Brazil nuts: and effective way to improve selenium status,* American Journal of Clinical Nutrition.

Tolman, D. (1998). Develop your Mental Muscle. Salem, Utah.

Tortura, G.J., Funke, B.R., Case, C.E. (1998). *Microbiology,* 6th ed. The Benjamin Cummings Publishing Company, Inc California. ISBN: 0805385355.

Turcotte, L.P., Kiens, B., and Richter, E.A. (1991). *Saturation kinetics of palmitate uptake in perfused skeletal muscle.* FEBS Letters.

Vargas, S., Romance, R., Petro, J.L., Bonilla, D.A., Galancho, I., Espinar, S., Kreider, R.B., Benítez-Porres, J. (2018). *Efficacy of ketogenic diet on body composition during resistance training in trained men: a randomized controlled trial.* Journal International Society Sports Nutrition. July.

Vukovich, M.D., Costill, D.L., Hickey, M.S., Trappe, S.W., Cole, K.J., Fink, W.J. (1993). *Effect of fat emulsion infusion and fat feeding on muscle glycogen utilization during cycle exercise.* Journal Applied Physiology.

Walker, N. (1970) *Fresh Vegetable and Fruit Juices: What's Missing in Your Body?* Prescott: Norwalk Press. ISBN: 0 89019 06704.

Wolfe, R.R., Klein, S., Carraro, F., Weber, J.M. (1990). *Role of triglyceride-fatty acid cycle in controlling fat metabolism in humans during and after exercise.* American Journal Physiology. (Endocrinol. Metab. 21).